brave parent

RAISING HEALTHY, HAPPY KIDS AGAINST ALL ODDS IN TODAY'S WORLD

DR. SUSAN MAPLES

burning soul press

praise for brave parent

"*In a society where parents may outlive their children due to endemic health issues, Brave Parent is a treasure trove of science, wisdom and support for parents wanting to guide their children into a life of health rather than disease. Dr Maples weaves an easy-to-read narrative through gut, brain and airway health, holding parents' hands with her practical tips and insights along the way because she knows, that it is the parents of the world that will set the future pathway for their children's health, with the right knowledge right at their fingertips.*"

Sharon Moore
Author of *Sleep-Wrecked Kids, helping parents raise happy, healthy kids, one sleep at a time*

"*Healthy habits in early childhood are the foundation for best health-related quality of life into old age. Dr Susan Maples has done a wonderful job researching the necessary building blocks and identifying a multitude of actions parents can take now to give their child advantages throughout life. I'm also in awe of her writing style. I only wish I had been able to read this when my own children were little!*"

Dr. Shereen Lim
Author of *Breathe, Sleep, Thrive: Discover how airway health can unlock your child's greater health, learning, and potential*

Every parent would benefit from reading Dr Susan Maples'
inspiring approachable book. There are so many easy to
implement suggestions. Your children will thank you.

Michael L Gelb DDS, MS
Co-Author of *Gasp: Airway Health, The Hidden Path to Wellness*

"I can't get enough of this book! It's comprehensive and so
compelling. Not only will you be hooked but as you read on
you will find answers to many questions you either didn't
know to ask, or know who to ask. This book is written from
the heart of a parent and the mind and expertise of an
accomplished (and ever curious) practitioner. It's a
tremendous resource covering everything from growth and
development to setting your child up for a lifetime of
healthy habits. This book will inspire, empower, and cheer
you on to make educated, healthy choices for your little
one."

Kelly Richardson
Author, Blogger, Pediatric Airway Health Advocate

This book is dedicated to my son, Hunter.
(You were so much fun to parent, honey. Thank you, from the bottom of my heart, for letting me tell your delightful and funny stories.)

And also to my other kids: my dear patients, nieces, nephews, and godchildren, especially: Michael Smallegan, Daniel Smallegan, Heather Oldani, Amber Oldani, Nichole Schiro, Ashlynn Schiro, Anthony Schiro, and my soul-daughter, Heather Baughman.

I wrote this book for you, so you might use my experience and research to raise happy, healthy kiddos of your own someday.

I love you all, with my whole heart.

Contents

CHAPTER 3: *digest*

SUPPORT THE BUGS IN YOUR KID'S GUT ... OR THEIR GUT WILL BUG THEM

CHAPTER 4: *breathe*

GROWING THE TONGUE BOX: IT'S THE SHAPE OF THINGS TO COME

CHAPTER 5: *sleep*   167
THE GREATEST UNDERRATED FRONTIER

CHAPTER 6: *feel and think*   205
BRAINIAC-YAK-YAK

CHAPTER 7: *chew and smile*

ORAL HEALTH WISE ... THE MOUTH IS A TATTLETALE

CHAPTER 8: *move* 305

FOSTERING A DAILY DOSE OF GET-UP-N-GO!

CHAPTER 9: *in closing* 335

GIDDYUP, YOU!

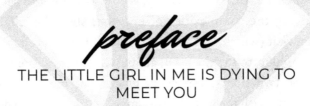

preface

THE LITTLE GIRL IN ME IS DYING TO MEET YOU

I'm often asked about how I got my motivation to write and speak about health throughout the world.

My health was given to me as an adolescent, a surprise from a brave stranger—a bonus Brave Parent, so to speak—on a random day in February 1972. Through my work as a health educator, motivator, and advocate, I'm paying my debt forward.

My story begins before birth. I grew weak lungs in the womb of a smoker. In 1959, when my brother Jim was four months old, my mom realized she was pregnant with me. She was freaking out, but her doctor reassured her that smoking more was a *good* way to relax anxious expectant mothers. (That's amazing to me.) In response, she doubled her smoking from one pack a day to two!

So, I was born, struggling for breath, to not one but two parents who smoked two packs a day each. In our little house there was at least one cigarette burning at all times, and in our car too. I spent my first few months in and out of the hospital's "oxygen tent" and the next twelve years in and out of doctors' offices. I developed chronic asthmatic bronchitis, exercise-induced asthma, and fifty-two environmental allergies, including grass, trees, weeds, pollen, and pets.

1

Often my disease would progress to pneumonia, which sent me back to the hospital. Finally, when I was twelve, my frustrated pediatrician gave up on my care. He recommended I see a specialist in adult internal medicine. Here's where my miracle begins.

Through professional friends, my mom found a young resident in internal medicine, Dr. Roberta Zapp, who was willing to see a child. After studying the complexities of my case, she scheduled a two-hour initial visit (which, by the way, wouldn't happen today).

I was nervous, to say the least, about what she was going to do to me in those two hours, especially given that my mom was not invited to come with me into the treatment room. Dr. Zapp walked in carrying my very thick medical chart. She introduced herself with a smile and then matter-of-factly plopped my chart on the counter. "Well, I've read this cover to cover, and it's a lot! I want to know what it's been like for *you*, living through all this."

I didn't know what to say. No one had ever asked me about *my story*. I also didn't understand why my thoughts would make any difference. Looking back, I realize that I responded like other chronically sick kids who have adapted to their illness, especially if it's the only life they've ever known. I didn't have much to say ... at first.

To encourage me, she asked good questions and I started to talk. With a chip on my shoulder, I told her the parts I hated about my life: I couldn't play outside without wheezing, couldn't do after-school activities because of my Monday and Thursday allergy shots, couldn't sleep at my girlfriend's house because they had feather pillows and a dog that I was allergic to.

I started to cry, and she just handed me a tissue and asked me another question. I went on through a stream of tears. I told her how I had become embarrassed to stand next to my peers because someone commented that I stink. (My clothes were laden with the scents of my vaporizer medicine and smoke.) I hated carrying an inhaler to gym class and often sitting out because of exercise-induced asthma. I grieved out loud that, in an effort to help my allergies, I had to get rid of my cats. And my dog. (Sob!) The more I talked, the more I cried, and Dr. Zapp just kept handing me tissues.

My indoor, sedentary home life had resulted in a bit of pre-adolescent weight gain and pre-diabetes. I endured that awful glucose tolerance test every year, waiting for the day I'd need insulin shots. The docs assumed my pre-diabetes was genetic because my paternal grandmother was diabetic. It was not!

I remember telling Dr. Zapp quite frankly that I was sick and tired of being sick and tired!

Hearing me, she held my gaze and let the silence linger for a minute. Then asked me one simple question: "What would you be willing to do if we could get rid of all your medications and all your allergies and help you live a normal life?"

"Like you could just do that!" I retorted with sarcastic doubt.

"I didn't say *I* could," she corrected me. "I asked what *you* would be willing to do if we could find a strategy to get you healthy without medication."

"I would do *anything,*" I said. I was hers!

"Great!" she replied. "I'll be right back."

She abruptly exited and closed the door behind her. Wiping my tears, I gathered my composure. She saw me. She heard me. And she had some ideas. I was beginning to feel the excitement of hope!

A few minutes later, she reentered and handed me a little piece of bubble wrap.

"Hold this!" she insisted. "Do you know what this is?" (It was 1972, and bubble wrap was a new technology.)

"I do!" I proclaimed. "We have some at home."

Then, like most kids would do, I pinched one of the little bubbles and made it pop. "Oh, don't pop that!" she warned. "Because every bubble counts! You see, this bubble plastic is just like your lungs. They are just like the little sacs that fill with air when you take a breath. They are called alveoli. And in the thin walls around each sac there are tiny circulating blood vessels called capillaries that pick up the oxygen out of each air sac and carry it to every other cell in your body. Without it you feel sick and tired."

She went on to explain, "Your lungs don't look like this, your air sacs aren't clear like these bubbles. They are full of fluid and pus. And the medications? They're just helping you expand those sacs so you can get more oxygen. Starting today, I'd like to see if we can train them to expand naturally, and slowly get you off all those medications."

Are you kidding me? That sounded too good to be true.

"What do I have to do?" I asked.

"A half hour of strenuous exercise a day."

With that, I was deflated. "I can't do it!" I confessed, "I can't even run for more than two minutes without a wheezing attack."

"Oh, honey, I know you can't ... *right now*," she said. "But I think if we work together, we could get you there."

I was all in, and that day we started to make a plan.

Dr. Zapp met with me once a week for six weeks, and then once a month for six months. She believed in me! And with her guidance and encouragement, I worked very hard. Within a month I joined a summer swim league. I remember staying in the slow lane, huffing and puffing my way through the workouts. Then six months later, I joined my high school swim team.

She also helped me stand up to my parents in an effort to avoid the smoke from their constantly lit cigarettes. (Remember that the concept of *secondhand smoke* wasn't even heard of back then.) Next, she encouraged me to clean up my diet. My mom let me help with grocery shopping, and I began substituting fruits and vegetables for ice cream and cookies.

Sure enough, as she'd set out to do, Dr. Zapp had delivered me from chronic illness to health in just three years. By fifteen, I was strong, lean, drug-free, allergy-free, and had no more threat of diabetes. I had become an athlete. I helped my high school swim team become state champions. Winning meant so much more than a trophy to me.

I'm writing this morning after my four-mile run. Daily exercise has long been my morning ritual. It helps keep me sane, strong, calm, lean, thinking clearly, and disease-free. Granted, Dr. Zapp didn't explain any of these attributes to me that day. She simply gave me what I needed to become the person I imagined I could be. And she started by listening to *my story*.

I learned on one blessed day the power a single adult can have on the life and health of another human being. And that lesson fuels my passion every single day. It's partly because of her that I'm a good doctor.

Dr. Zapp is a perfect example of how a Brave Parent doesn't have to be the birth parent at all—it can be anyone who *sees* that child's wellness better than they can at any given moment. With my own child I continually prayed for adults who would see the best in him and conspire for his best interest despite societal norms, expectations, or fear of crossing the line and gaining a one-star review on Facebook. A Brave Parent is one who is willing to empower children to make choices that best serve their long-term health and capabilities—and *not* to make choices that feed their detrimental, short-lived gratifications.

I have come to learn that *lifespan* and *healthspan* are two very different things. Unhealthy adulthood began in childhood.

Often our greatest challenges morph into our most precious gifts. I have experienced myself how a child can take the driver's seat for a lifetime of health. I am passionate about helping you teach your children how to drive, navigate, avoid potholes, and avert life-threatening obstacles. I hope the nuggets you need in this book serendipitously appear and that it helps you do just that.

I offer my blessings to you and your sweet children!

introduction

A DOSE OF TODAY'S REALITY: IT'S ENOUGH TO MAKE YOU CRY

"Healthy citizens are the greatest asset any country can have."
-Winston Churchill 1874–1965

"Healthy children are the greatest asset any family can have."
-(My version)

U nfortunately, health often goes unappreciated until we're in crisis.

Speaking of crisis ... as I write this, the health of our country is in serious jeopardy, and it happened on my watch, as a health care professional. It clearly wasn't the case when I began my career in dentistry only thirty-six years ago. It should disturb us all that the US measures as the *sickest* population among industrialized (OECD) countries and at more than double the cost of care of *any* other country.

As a whole, we are heavier, more diseased, more medicated, slower moving, faster paced, more socially pressured, less satisfied, more anxious, and more depressed than ever! And it's not about to stop. By 2050, it's projected that 43% of us will suffer from obesity, half from heart disease, half from cancer, one-third from type 2 diabetes, and 40% from anxiety disorder.

Wouldn't it be nice if *your* kids were the exception to these skyrocketing disease trends? And if *they* drove change among their peers?

I wholeheartedly believe if we are ever going to change this abysmal situation, we must do it through a generation of children who "get it." You, as the bravest of Brave Parents, can ensure this by working together to change detrimental habits during your kid's formative years. Stand tall against cultural norms. Refuse to be intimidated. Are you ready? Just read on ... with a curious and open mind.

Throughout the book, I use the word *parent* to include any brave adult who loves and cares for a growing child. Even if you're not caring for children in your immediate household, keep reading. After all, there's no such thing as other people's children when we're all facing this health crisis together.

A WAKE-UP CALL

In late winter of 2020, every US citizen stepped into freak mode. We began to face COVID-19, a pernicious virus that could potentially wipe out 1–2% of our population. Our immediate future looked like a horror movie.

So, imagine my surprise on March 2, 2020, when I turned on the morning news to get a panic-pulse on the imploding pandemic, and the terrifying report was interrupted by a cheery-voiced newscaster chortling, "On a brighter note, today is National Egg McMuffin Day, and McDonald's is giving away Egg McMuffins for breakfast. Also, Wendy's launched its new breakfast menu ... *and* KFC is highlighting its new breakfast sandwich: two glazed donuts with hand-breaded extra crispy fried chicken in between."

66

... medicine has been on a quest to **treat one problem** at a time, prescribing drugs only to **quell the symptoms**, not the disease itself.

The system is *broken!*

Imagine instead, all health care professionals taking time to identify the **underlying root cause of disease** and learn to effectively facilitate behavior change.

Talk about a *revolution.*

99

Are you kidding me?! The irony was too much! Please "get it" that the death toll from our collection of lifestyle-related, *noncommunicable diseases* (NCDs) is astronomically greater than the pernicious coronavirus ever hoped to be. Eating commercialized, processed food is a slow-kill, so we are desensitized and dull to it. By the way, when did we give McDonald's its own holiday?

I heard over and over that COVID-19 was even killing young,

healthy people. I was quick to suggest that *young* and *healthy* are not synonymous. The majority of children in our culture are suffering from any number of lifestyle-related conditions: obesity, insulin resistance, nonalcoholic fatty liver disease, early cardiovascular inflammation, active caries disease (rampant tooth decay), and addiction to everything from caffeine and sugar to heroin.

It's estimated that 75% of our country's health expenditure is for these lifestyle diseases that are *preventable*. Shouldn't it scare us that every forty seconds one American dies of a heart attack and every four minutes another by stroke? Yet cardiovascular disease is preventable altogether if we would just eat real food, move more, and sleep well.

Here's another serious issue. Our health care system doesn't pay for prevention, only treatment. Recognize that "preventive" procedures like colonoscopy, mammography, and PSA tests (screen for prostate cancer) are for early detection, *not* prevention. We need medical coverage for all aspects of teaching how to live a healthy lifestyle. And we need to revamp our processed food supply.

Instead, medicine has been on a quest to treat one problem at a time, prescribing drugs only to quell the symptoms, *not* the disease itself. The system is broken! Imagine instead, all health care professionals taking time to identify the underlying root cause of disease and learn to effectively facilitate behavior change. Talk about a revolution.

To do that we must learn to see the human body as a whole—and learn what to do to care for it. How do we breathe? What's the quality and quantity of our sleep? What do we eat? How do we effectively move our bodies? How do we respond to stress, both acute and chronic? How do we nourish and nurture our brains? And how do we improve our gut/mouth microbiome?

YOUR BRAVE PARENT JOURNEY BEGINS NOW!

If you want to help put a child in the driver's seat on a lifelong journey to health, consider this book your roadmap. Let me help you set up your kiddo for a lifetime of health—truly *against all odds* in today's world.

BRAVE PARENT DISCLAIMERS

I'M NOT YOUR DOC

This is indeed an evidence-based book. But the information contained in these topics is not intended nor implied to be a substitute for professional medical advice; it is provided for educational purposes only. You assume full responsibility for how you choose to use this information.

Always seek the advice of your physician, dentist, or other qualified healthcare providers before starting any new treatment or discontinuing an existing treatment. Talk with them about any questions you may have regarding your child's medical condition(s).

The information and materials presented in *Brave Parent* are meant to supplement the information that you obtain from your health care providers. Nothing contained in these topics is intended to be used for medical diagnosis or treatment.

If there is a disagreement between the information presented herein and what your health care provider has told you—it is best to follow their guidance.

I'M PRONOUN-BEFUDDLED!

We are amidst a huge cultural shift in language that honors all people, regardless of their identified gender. As a late baby boomer, this was not a challenge I had to face in my earlier writing. Throughout the book, however, I have wholeheartedly wanted to include all people, respect all people, and help all people, regardless of their gender identity, skin color, belief systems, or political affiliation. This is a book about HEALTH, which I want for YOU and your children.

In trying to be inclusive, I have come to realize that many languages, including English, do not have a gender-neutral or third-gender pronoun list available. Also, the dichotomy of "he and she" in English does not leave room for other gender identities, which is a source of frustration to the transgender and genderqueer communities.

Please give me grace as I included *all* pronouns throughout the book. I, too, am a work in progress.

FOR PARENTS OF SPECIAL NEEDS KIDS

You are a small but mighty audience, and I want to champion you for your extra special bravery. Many of my favorite patients are special needs children.

One of my closest friends is a global leader in the medical care of children with disabilities, so I consulted her on what message I might include specific to your kiddos. After reading *Brave Parent*, she said this:

"Children with disabilities need to stay healthy and strong just like every other child, and sometimes that can be a challenge because they may have trouble moving. This can lead to problems with digestion and constipation, but the dietary advice in the Eat chapter can help parents tackle that problem and keep things humming along. In fact, the entire book is filled with great nuggets of information that I will definitely share with the families I care for in my practice. I loved this book and wish I had it when my kids were little!"

- Dr. Lisa Thornton, Division Chief for Pediatric Rehabilitation Medicine, Sidra Medicine, and Assistant Clinical Professor of Pediatrics Weill Cornell Medicine Qatar

The Brave Parent journey is personal for everyone, and not for the faint of heart. I stand in awe of you, as your challenges are much more complicated. My heart is with you as I write these pages.

CHAPTER ONE

eat

YOUR KID VERSUS TODAY'S FOOD CRAZINESS: IT'S A LOT TO SWALLOW

INTRODUCTION

How did it happen that the still-climbing prevalence of overweight or obesity has grown to 55% of US adults and 30% of US kids?

You know the answer. Most of our individual food pantries and refrigerators are a hot mess. The biggest culprit is the processing and commercialization of our food supply. We each make about 250 food decisions EVERY day, and somehow, we've lost our way. You might not be surprised to learn that among the US top fifty consumed foods there isn't a single piece of produce—unless you count french fries or potato chips.

I believe it would help immeasurably if our food manufacturers all agreed to overhaul our food supply, replacing inherently dangerous foods with healthy ones. But that's not happening anytime soon. They are in fierce competition, only to earn the attention of your tastebuds ... oh, and the dollars in your bank account.

In the 200,000-year history of our human race, it's been in the blink of an eye—only about forty-five years—that our people grew to be fat and sick from this massive change in lifestyle.

As frustrating as that might be, it's next to impossible for us, as individuals, to influence public policy toward such a cleanup, and trust me, it's also missing from the agenda of either political party.

Wreaking havoc with the ever-profitable conglomerates of big food, big pharma, big distilleries, lobbyists, and even modern medicine is apparently un-American. By the way, I'm not nearly as brave in discussing this debacle as my friend Dr. Robert Lustig, who just penned the brilliant book *Metabolical: The Lure and the Lies of Processed Food, Nutrition, and Modern Medicine*. If you haven't yet read it, put it very next on your list!

The bottom line: don't hold your breath for policy change. Instead, we will need to tackle this catastrophe as a grass roots effort ... one child at a time, one Brave Parent at a time.

Our responsibility as Brave Parents is to provide healthy and appetizing foods for our children. Their job is to eat them when they're hungry.

Our grocery store food supply is not our only problem, however. Our *mindset* around *dieting* is a jumble! Fifty-seven percent of US women are dieting as you read this. We are preoccupied and super confused about what to eat, what not to eat, and when to eat in order to lose weight. Over the past two decades the diet industry has tripled its gross annual revenues to over sixty *billion* dollars! This reflects a culture that has developed mighty unhealthful relationships with food.

This section is about all of this: what to eat, what not to eat, and how to help your child develop positive, healthful relationships with food. I know you can do this! Let's start in the very beginning.

66 Our responsibility as

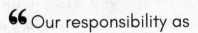

is to provide healthy
and appetizing foods
for our children.

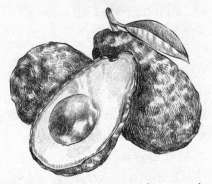

Their job is to eat them when
they're hungry. **99**

1.1 A DIET-CRAZED COUNTRY

We are born with an amazing innate ability to balance and regulate our energy intake to serve our bodies well on any given day. We seek food when we're hungry, and we don't when we're not. A simple feedback loop, right? That's how our bodies were designed, but our intake of processed food has broken that feedback loop. Now many of us eat because food is available and stop when it's gone, with no ability to self-regulate. That's when we get in trouble with metabolic disease.

Losing our innate ability to regulate our ideal caloric intake happens gradually. How our hunger-feeding circuitry becomes increasingly muted is multifaceted and complicated—and the fix isn't easy either. Let me help debunk this phenomenon for you in the pages ahead.

The fact that you're reading a book on children's health means you've probably already grappled with your own understanding of which foods are inherently "good" and "bad." Most of us keep an angel perched on one shoulder and devil on the other, each battling over our willpower. This may leave us eating somewhere between a green smoothie with flax meal (declaring, "Okay, that didn't taste too bad.") and a sleeve of Oreo cookies ("That was yummy, but now I'm guilty, ashamed, and feel like crap."). We have demonized some foods and glorified others—often without scientific basis.

Many of us can't quite figure out how to achieve and maintain a lower weight, and we blame ourselves. Sometimes our guilt starts gnawing at us, and we opt for a hard reset—we adopt a fad diet designed to help us lose weight and feel better.

I bet you already know that the perfect diet plan doesn't exist! It doesn't matter if it's ketogenic, dairy-free, low-carb, vegan, vegetarian, paleo, pescatarian, lectin-free, grain-free, intermittent fasting, blood typing ... the very idea of a "diet" is flawed.

66

We tend not to force our children to follow our new diet, but **beware**... our kids are watching us, and they're **modeling our behavior.**

It's true that their **relationships to food** are forever **influenced** by witnessing our beliefs, behaviors, and patterns.

And we can *do better*.

99

Let's make it personal. Most of us have explored at least one of these diet plans. We usually begin with an almost fanatical zeal—and our enthusiasm calls others onto the bandwagon. With each of these, the weight loss works right at first, doesn't it? Then we somehow fall off, and the rebound often leaves us even less energized and heavier than when we started.

Many scientists indict the fad diet culture as the most powerful obstacle to achieving optimal health. When we dive into a new diet that promises to wipe out our belly fat or eradicate our chronic inflammation, we buy it, hook, line, and sinker! And when we fail, we blame ourselves, not the diet. That's a perfect setup to create powerfully heightened negative emotions toward food in general. If you are a serial dieter, you no-doubt already realize it's a no-win lifestyle.

We tend not to force our children to follow our new diet, but beware ... our kids are watching us, and they're modeling our behavior. It's true that their relationships to food are forever influenced by witnessing *our* beliefs, behaviors, and patterns. And we can do better.

During my pregnancy with Hunter, I met a brilliant Michigan State University professor named Dr. Esther Parks. She was speaking at a dental conference about recognizing eating disorders. In her presentation, she projected a slide of the timeline continuum from normal eating (birth) to pathologic (or unhealthy) eating. I was shocked to learn that that when we become a chronic dieter, we have already crossed the line between normal eating and pathologic eating. The slope from chronic dieting to anorexia or bulimia is a slippery one. It's all about seeking more and more control. More on that ahead in section 1.5 of this chapter.

She further described her therapies for people with eating disorders, helping them reestablish a heathy relationship to food. After the Q&A, I rushed to the stage to ask her if I could hire her as my personal consultant. I wanted desperately to know how to raise my soon-to-be-born child to become a healthy eater from the start. In that moment, it seemed like that just might be the holy grail for raising a happy, healthy kid. What I learned from Dr. Parks became the scaffold for the Eight Food Pillars you will discover beginning in section 1.3.

1.2 CHRONIC INFLAMMATION FROM FOOD

Inflammation has become a big buzzword in the health literacy world. The literature on the role of inflammation on health has grown exponentially over the past few decades. I believe it's still poorly understood, so let's start there.

Acute inflammation is a good thing! It helps keep us alive. In response to injury or infection, our immune system signals an immediate response, sending helper cells (white blood cells) to clean up and repair the site. Think of a small paper cut on your finger. As soon as you experience that initial sting, the skin around the cut begins to turn red, swell, and generate heat. That's the result of your capillaries opening up, like a big highway, transporting a truckload of blood cells (such as macrophages) to gobble up the invading bacteria, clot the bleeding, and initiate the healing process. Macrophages produce *cytokines*, a collection of chemical communicators that signal the need to recruit more (or less) help.

Acute inflammation means that it's relatively short-lived. Thus, the infection or injury is resolved within days to weeks, and the inflammation goes away.

But what if the inflammation never goes away? What if the cytokines stay elevated in response to a never-ending source of insult? That is called *chronic inflammation*, and it spells trouble with a capital *T*.

Chronic inflammation causes the lining of *all* your blood vessels to erode. The lining is called *endothelium*; it's only ten to sixteen cell layers thick and in constant repair. Flaws in the endothelium allow bad stuff (bacteria with its macrophages) and small dense fat droplets (blood lipids called LDLs) to enter and multiply or collect inside the blood vessel walls. Many refer to this as a "plaque." This is how chronic systemic inflammation (CSI) is at the root cause of our number one disease, cardiovascular (heart) disease. If you want to learn more, I encourage you to read *Beat the Heart Attack Gene*, written by two brilliant scientists and teachers, Bradley Bale, MD, and Amy Doneen, ARNP.

Chronic inflammation in the body has many possible causes, like the smoldering infection of gum disease and *noninfectious* conditions such as obesity, insulin resistance, and arthritis.

Food sensitivities can also cause CSI, just as they stimulate dysfunction and discomfort in your gut and mouth. Think again of your response to a paper cut and imagine it on the widespread geography of your gut lining.

This gets more confusing when I explain that you don't need specific food sensitivities to develop CSI from food. It turns out that processed food does that all by itself. It's less about the food and more about the way it was processed, including preservatives, flavor enhancers, sweeteners, thickeners, coloring agents, and other added toxins. The difference between a Dorito and a Frito is shocking. A Frito, while certainly not the healthiest food on the planet, has only three ingredients: corn, oil, and salt. A Dorito has more than forty-four. It's hard to know the exact number since some of the chemicals listed are proprietary blends and their true makeup is undisclosed. I'm not trying to demonize any particular "food" but only to create a healthy respect for the added work it takes your body to clean up the chemical spill caused from just one chip.

If you are going to keep eating processed foods, download the smartphone app called Fooducate, which allows you to scan the bar code on your grocery items to get a letter grade on its health value. It also lets you click on "alternatives" to see any similar foods that have a better letter grade. Fooducate provides explanations and nutrition info, too, but even if you don't have time, it's a quick and easy helper while you're grocery shopping.

We teach our adolescent patients to use the app and encourage them to go through their cupboards and fridge, scanning their favorite products, recording healthier substitutes. The assignment is to make a newly revised shopping list for whomever does the household grocery shopping.

" If you are going to keep eating **processed foods**, download the smartphone app called **Fooducate**, which allows you to **scan** the bar code on your **grocery items** to get a letter **grade** on its *health value*. **"**

A more advanced guide is the Dietary Inflammatory Index (DII) which was developed to measure the role of diet in relation to signs and symptoms of CSI. The DII debuted in 2009, based on 927 peer-reviewed articles that linked any aspect of diet to elevated blood inflammatory biomarkers (IL-1β, IL-4, IL-6, IL-10, TNF-α, and hs-CRP). The newest revised index included another 127 peer-reviewed articles. The index is rather complex and nuanced, but I'm hopeful this will become more user-friendly and better known in the years ahead.

Some conditions associated with a pro-inflammatory diet as scored by the DII are cardiovascular disease (CVD), chronic obstructive pulmonary disease (COPD), arthritis (both rheumatoid and osteoarthritis), gut dysbiosis (a bacterial imbalance resulting in a host of wretched GI symptoms), irritable bowel syndrome and disease, ulcerative colitis, and Crohn's disease.

If you're interested in creating an anti-inflammatory nutrition regimen for you and your children, look at the principles of the Mediterranean diet. It's the most widely studied because the

Mediterranean region of the world has a well-studied population with the least dietary inflammation. This diet is low in sugar and has a broad range of vegetables, fruits, nuts, legumes, healthy fats, and whole grains. It's also considered the easiest to sustain because we don't have to deprive ourselves of any one macronutrient. Plus, many of us already enjoy Mediterranean foods. The only problem is it requires some food prep. All anti-inflammatory diets eliminate virtually all the "convenient" foods you might get from a fast-food window or grocery store prepackaged options.

1.3 INTRODUCING THE EIGHT MOST PRACTICAL FOOD PILLARS FOR KIDS

As a Brave Parent, it's time to build healthy relationships with food to foster lifelong eating practices for kids! The *Eight Food Pillars* that follow were developed to help kiddos keep (or regain) their natural hunger acumen and to appreciate healthy food.

After all these years, I still pass on much of Esther Parks's advice to my parents of infants. I have interwoven my insights with Esther's in order to keep pace with contemporary trends—most especially the massive increase in sugar consumption from 1993 till now. All medical and dental associations alike have issued warnings to eliminate liquid sugar from your child's diet. And *breakfast* has turned into dessert-fest with the amount of added sugar food manufacturers pour into everything from yogurt to smoothies and certainly breakfast cereals.

It's time to draw some lines and focus on a new respect for our bodies and their yearning for *real* food. I can tell you from my own experience in raising Hunter and from witnessing these rules in action with countless patients over the years, these simple rules work!

As you consider each, keep in mind that they are not just for the littles of your household. These are pillars for *everyone* in the family including tweens, teens, and yes, YOU! Why? Because your health matters, and because children do as you do ... not as you say.

Pillar #1: Never Force or Restrict Food

Children's bodies function exquisitely to regulate their intake until we as adults wreak havoc with that. Here's how we do it. Starting from infancy, kids will eat according to their own variable energy needs—as they should. Some days they're so hungry we feel guilty feeding them so much. Other days they barely touch their food, and it worries us. If you're like me, the latter actually concerns you more because it feels so gratifying to feed your kiddos.

So, we start to condition them to override their hunger and eat what we ask of them. We train them into eating "regular meals" of our choosing, routinizing their food intake, no matter what their energy needs are. We want them to be more like most US adults, who have long lost their ability to discern their own hunger.

The hypothalamus is a region of the brain that controls satiety (satisfaction) and feeding (appetite). The two most significant hormones that help regulate this energy balance are leptin and ghrelin. When we screw up this natural system, it's hard to get it back. Forcing and restricting food is not the whole problem—you'll read more about these brain-players in the chapters on Breathe and Sleep —but your response to their variable appetite does play a significant role.

We commonly tell children they can't have dessert unless they finish eating what's on their dinner plate. Instead, try honoring their current appetite. On days when you have planned a desert, if you notice your child is not eating much, serve an equally small portion of dessert.

Trust that the brain and responding hormones are much more astute at food regulation than you are. You'll get less freaked out by your children's variable food consumption.

Pillar #2: Don't Use Food as a Reward or Punishment

Rewards, punishments, and bribery are all so common in parenting. I get it, but try not to use food as your bargaining chip. Avoid offers like "If you eat your asparagus, you can have a Popsicle." Or "Wait ... you *can't* eat that cookie ... because you haven't cleaned your room yet."

Keep in mind that it's up to you to convey the purpose of food—to nourish our bodies, *not* to earn extrinsic rewards or garnish penalties.

In my dental office I have many times heard a parent negotiating with their child, that if they are brave while getting a filling (on a decayed tooth from a sugar habit), they'll take them for ice cream or a Slurpee right after. (Are you kidding me right now?)

So, when you do resort to bribery (because, let's face it, we all do it), try not to glorify unhealthy foods or drinks. In fact, think about other-than-food rewards such as storytelling time, a nature hike, a craft project, playing a favorite game, or a back rub.

Pillar #3: Enforce the "Polite Bite"

Our brains have an amazing way of adopting preferences around the foods we habitually eat. It's the gift of *neuroplasticity*, the ability of the brain to reorganize and change activity in response to changing stimuli.

Most people don't know it takes an average of *seven* tastes of a food for our brains to switch from a once-disliked food to an *acceptable* and then a *preferable* food. So, if we establish an agreement in our homes that *everyone* (adults and kids alike) must taste *everything* on their plate, kids will cultivate a broader—and therefore healthier —palate.

There is a caveat to this rule. Seven tastes are an *average*, but we tend to like sweet foods more quickly, with savory foods taking longer. Kids get this rule easily and will continue to taste foods, losing track of the number of times they've tried it.

"So, when you do **resort to bribery** (because, let's face it, we all do it), try **not to glorify unhealthy foods or drinks.** In fact, think about **other-than-food** *rewards* such as storytelling time, a nature hike, a craft project, playing a favorite game, or a back rub. **"**

I remember when I served my nephew and son (both four years old at the time) a hot porridge, called Cream of Wheat, for breakfast. It was prepared with a pinch of salt and a bit of whole milk and served with a pat of melting butter on top. Daniel turned his nose up, and Hunter enthusiastically encouraged him to try it. (It was his favorite. He called it "wumpy cereal" because he liked it lumpy.) Daniel cautiously took a taste and immediately spit it out with a "Yuck!" Hunter replied just as enthusiastically, "It's okay Daniel. Just take six more bites, and you'll like it!" I had to laugh as I explained that it doesn't work if you take all seven bites the same day.

Keep in mind that some foods incite a noxious response, so don't force a child to swallow a food. If your child gags at the taste of noxious foods, they can taste it over the sink and spit it out. What's most important is that the brain registers the taste.

Some call this the "no-thank-you bite." I prefer to call this the *polite bite* because it also honors the cook (even if it's in a restaurant), who took the time to prepare and serve each part of the meal.

Pillar #4: The One-Finger Rule

This is perfect for a toddler who is sitting in the front seat of your grocery cart. When you're buying packaged foods, if your child can't cover the ingredient list with one finger, that food simply doesn't earn its way into your grocery cart. Esther taught me this twenty-eight years ago, but today some of the ingredient lists are printed in minuscule fonts. So as soon as your child can count, you can modify this rule to ditch commercial foods that have more than five ingredients, especially if they don't sound like real food.

Consistently inspecting the ingredient lists is a good way to cultivate your kiddo's curiosity about what ingredients we are putting in our bodies. If there is *anything* on the list that sounds foreign to you—less like real food and more like a chemical additive—take a minute to google it. You both might be grossed out about additives that make this "food" not really food at all.

> **66** It's not that **sugar** is inherently bad because every **human cell** requires some for **energy.** But, unless you're wrestling a gorilla or running a marathon, a little goes a *long way.* **99**

Pillar #5: Eliminate All Sugary Beverages (Including Fruit Juice) from Your Home

Purge them all. This includes fruit juice, sports drinks, sweetened water, sweet tea, soda (of course), and energy drinks.

This is an added rule (not an Esther-rule) because sugar consumption has risen ridiculously since Dr. Esther Parks counseled me—and about *half* of our kids' sugar intake is reportedly from sugar-sweetened beverages (SSBs). This includes any beverages sweetened with any kind of sugar or nonnutritive sweeteners (NNSs).

When children start to prefer fruit juice to water and milk, it predisposes them to wanting sports drinks, the highly addictive sodas, and energy drinks. Because drinks are so important, they get their own chapter, and we will dive deeper into NNSs there.

By now it's no secret that I view our crazy sugar consumption as the root of all evil when it comes to obesity and metabolic disease stimulus. It's not that sugar is inherently bad because every human cell requires some for energy. But, unless you're wrestling a gorilla or running a marathon, a little goes a long way. It's the amount, the kind of sugar, and how fast it gets into your bloodstream that has the potential to drive disease. In chronic excess, sugar is dangerous! It leads to fat storage and *insulin resistance*—an inflammatory condition that spirals downward to type 2 diabetes.

There's another disease that's sugar-driven, especially from SSBs, and it has nothing to do with metabolic syndrome. It's the number one, most prevalent disease among humans including all ages, geographic locations, and demographics. Can you guess it? Dental Caries (the disease of tooth decay)—and believe it or not, it's 100% preventable. (See chapter 7 Chew and Smile.)

But that's not the only *preventable* disease that excess sugar consumption has been implicated in. Let's include 90% of obesity, cardiovascular disease, type 2 diabetes, hypertension, cognitive decline, cancer, and nonalcoholic fatty liver disease (NAFLD) to name just a few.

As Brave Parents you must live by all these pillars as well because little eyes are watching you with admiration and envy. So, clean your cupboards and fridge by eliminating *all* SSBs for you and your children.

Pillar #6: Leave Sweetened Cereals in the Store

By now, you know I'm not a fan of most processed foods, let alone candied-up breakfast cereals. Beginning your child's day with a bowl full of sugar makes for an abysmal start. Try cooking a whole grain porridge such as oatmeal or Cream of Wheat and sweeten it with bananas or berries. If you're determined to shop the cereal aisle, at least buy unsweetened cereals such as Bran Flakes, Corn Flakes, Rice Krispies, Cheerios, or Grape Nuts. Add fruit for a sweeter taste.

What if your kids are already hooked on sugared-up cereals and you're not ready to cook their breakfast? Buy a box of unsweetened cereal and put the old-fashioned sugar bowl back on the table for a while. Let your kiddos sweeten it themselves. If you're a grandparent, this might be a flashback to your youth. Before the food manufacturers laced 75% of their products with sugar, we all had a sugar bowl with a teaspoon in it, sitting right next to the salt and pepper on the table. These were condiments. Even with a bottomless sugar bowl in front of your children, there is no way they can add as much sugar to the bowl as the food manufacturers do!

Getting rid of sugary breakfast foods won't just protect your child's insulin sensitivity but your wallet as well.

If your kids complain, explain. Be brave! Don't give in! Tell them how much you love them and how much their health and happiness mean to you. I promise you the healthy breakfast foods you choose will become their favorites in no time at all. We can always count on the brain to re-wire our preferences around what we habitually eat. This concept is called neuroplasticity, and I'll describe it in greater detail in section 6.9.

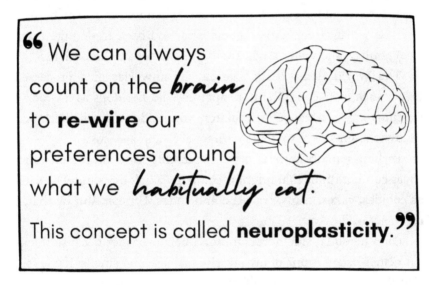

> " We can always count on the *brain* to **re-wire** our preferences around what we *habitually eat.* This concept is called **neuroplasticity.** "

Pillar #7: Eat Whole Foods

Whole foods are foods that are unprocessed and refined as little as possible. They are in the form most resembling their natural source. This rule is a big one. It means truly avoiding manufactured food.

When you hear the term *whole foods,* people are generally talking about a plant-based diet such as fruits, vegetables, whole grains, tubers, and legumes. More on that in the next pillar. Meanwhile, most families still eat meat and fish. If you do, try to ensure that they are also unprocessed and raised healthily and humanely.

Why humanely? Imagine being a cow, chicken, or pig ... a "farm" animal who is raised in a feedlot rather than on a farm. This animal lives his life indoors—he never sees sunlight, never gets to eat a blade of grass, can't even take a step on his own—and if that's not enough, he's continually pumped full of hormones and antibiotics to fatten him up for slaughter as young as possible. That's not humane. But it's not his psyche I'm worried about. I'm clearly describing a sick animal—an animal you should definitely *not* eat.

To make matters worse, grasp that all the toxins he accumulates in his fat are passed right through to us when we eat it. The bottom line? Seek drug-free, 100% organic grass-fed beef, free-range (cage free) poultry, and wild-caught (not farm-raised) smallmouth fish.

The World Health Organization has now classified processed meats such as bacon, salami, pepperoni, and hot dogs as a Group 1 Carcinogen. As a cancer stimulator, your kiddo's fresh deli meat sandwich ranks right up there with tobacco and asbestos.

Perhaps equally harmful is the exhausting list of processed flour-sugar combinations that might accompany a baloney sandwich such as cookies, cakes, chips, crackers, and sodas. Unreal! And by that, I mean *not real*!

On a personal side note, I'm not a bacon-basher because thick-cut rasher bacon is one of my favorite tastes ... and smells. If you feel that way, too, these kinds of meats should be purchased *uncured*, eaten in small quantities, and only on occasion. Moderation is key in all your guilty food pleasures.

If you haven't yet attained a copy of Michael Pollan's book *Food Rules*, get that. My patients love it because it's simple, smart, and fun to read as a family. It's chock-full of memes like, "If it came from a plant, eat it; if it was made in a plant, don't."

Pillar #8: Eat More Plants than Animals, Especially Plants with Color

The vast majority of health experts consider a plant-based diet the healthiest choice to prevent systemic inflammation. The majority of Americans live on the opposite end of this spectrum, favoring meats, cheeses, and processed carbs.

Did you know that *FIBER is universally considered our number one nutrient deficiency?* Fiber significantly slows the absorption of sugar into our bloodstream, thereby controlling the insulin release and protecting our innate insulin *sensitivity.*

If I lost you there, just know that increasing fiber will help you and your children decrease the risk of metabolic disease including type 2 diabetes, plus help avoid heart attack and stroke in the future as well. As for today? A high fiber diet is important for weight control, digestion (gut health), and elimination (regular and healthy poops). I trained Hunter to see his poops as a measure of health, aiming for foot-long floaters, which we lightheartedly called FLFs. If you do this, don't be surprised when you're summoned into the bathroom for a proud moment before the toilet gets flushed. (Don't worry, FLF-bragging should end sometime before high school graduation. LOL)

Only 24% of Americans eat the minimal recommendation of five half-cup servings a day of vegetables and fruit. That's incredibly sad. Remember that we need both *soluble* fiber and *insoluble* fiber ... and we get *both* from vegetables, fruits, nuts, and whole grains. Plants also contain *phyto*nutrients, antioxidants, and anti-inflammatory chemicals that boost cell health.

We need to be mindful of herbicides and pesticides, but organic produce is significantly more expensive. Consider adhering to the *Clean Fifteen* and the *Dirty Dozen.* The Clean Fifteen is a searchable list of plants that are safe to eat without being organically grown, and the Dirty Dozen is a list of those that aren't.

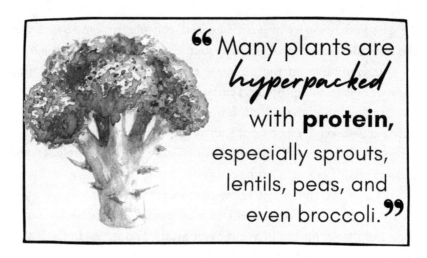

> **"Many plants are** *hyperpacked* **with protein,** especially sprouts, lentils, peas, and even broccoli.**"**

Many people worry that a plant-based diet will leave them protein deficient. It is simply not the case. Many plants are hyper-packed with protein, especially sprouts, lentils, peas, and even broccoli. If you are going to keep meat and fish in your family's diet, consider designating it as the garnish on the plate, not the mainstay. This is not only the healthiest choice but the most economical. While you will pay more for higher quality meat, you will be consuming less of it.

If your kids don't enjoy veggies and fruits, you can change that. Frequency invites preference! Include a variety of them at every meal and reinforce the *polite bite.* Here's a tip: leave a big fruit and veggie bowl out on the kitchen counter for easy grazing. Plus, whenever kids are hanging around, cut the fruits and veggies into finger food for snacking convenience.

Another tip: when prepping fruits and veggies, be sure to bag individual servings to drop into their school lunch bag. Leftover grilled veggies make a great snack or lunch addition too.

Stay with it and one day very soon, you'll see the rewards of your efforts. I remember getting an email from my son's sixth grade principal after eating lunch next to him. He was shocked to see Hunter open a ziplock bag of baby spinach and happily munch it down. In disbelief, he had to ask Hunter what he was eating. Hunter said, "You don't recognize spinach, Dr. Tweedy? It's delicious, do you want to try it?" Dr. Tweedy replied, "I thought that's what I saw. Next you'll probably tell me you like brussels sprouts too." And I about lost my lunch as Hunter reached in his brown bag and pulled out a bag of roasted brussels declaring, "These are my favorite, and I love when we have leftovers from dinner!"

1.4 CREATING A WONDERFUL DINNER EXPERIENCE

Have you ever driven through a fast-food window and tossed the bag in the back seat for your children to scarf down on the way to a dance class or sports practice? I have! And I hated it. The things we rush through in life, just to get them over with, are things we don't value. In our crazy, harried lives we often rush through mealtime, giving kids the subtle but distinct message that we don't value it.

There is sanctity in eating nutritious, delicious meals and enjoying them together. Preparing for that takes time and effort, and it's important. It's not convenient, but it's important! Teaching our kids to *value* the effort it takes to feed your body well takes as much training as learning to shop for and prepare the nutritious foods.

Try creating a dinnertime ritual, where your beloveds are invited to the table, but their cell phones or television programs are not. For Hunter, I was committed to creating a feeling of celebration by routinely using cloth napkins at dinner (easily dropped into the washing machine during table clearing), setting the silverware properly, and always lighting a (scentless) candle or two in the middle of the table. While some might view that as formal or fussy, I saw it as creating a sacred space of sorts, to honor the food, conversation, and our fellowship.

I was particularly aware of my responsibility to teach Hunter how to feed himself well, over a lifetime. Preparing food is definitely not a gender-specific duty, but I still witness our culture as one that emphasizes a female's affinity for the kitchen over a male's. When I ask a man if he cooks, I often get the response, "Well, I man the grill. Does that count?"

Because I love cooking, I'm efficient at it and enjoy serving people. I had to force myself to share that responsibility with Hunter. He had another challenge. In middle school and high school, he was a three-sport athlete, a pianist, and a high-achiever in academics. He had even less unstructured time at home than I did. So, one of the ways I prepared him to be a good cook later in life was to teach foundations of cooking well. I don't believe we need formal recipes to be a good cook. If we learn instinctively how to combine fresh foods, herbs, and spices we enjoy, it will taste great 95% of the time. That means we need to learn how to recognize the tastes of specific ingredients.

I made a game of it with Hunter. Upon his first bite of a food, I would challenge him to identify just what he was seeing and tasting on his fork. He learned to identify a myriad of whole grains and vegetables, meats and seafoods, and cheeses. Next, the tougher subtle hints of spices and herbs. Occasionally I had him try a single (fresh) herb, so he could eventually tease out the tastes and aromas of parsley, dill, garlic, rosemary, cilantro, basil, lemon balm, oregano, etc. Spices were the trickiest. It's easy to tell the difference between cinnamon and nutmeg, but much harder to discern the difference between red pepper flakes, cayenne, and white pepper.

For us, because cell phones, computers, and TV-watching were never part of our dinner time, that notion was never challenged. If technology has already invaded your dinner table, talk about what you might gain from an unplugged dinner hour and try forging some new agreements around it. Make it fun and impactful. If you can't think of creative ways to do that, there are lots of fun card deck conversation starters to stimulate humorous, educational, brave, and vulnerable dialogue.

One last piece of advice. Continue to remind each other to eat slowly and mindfully until it becomes a habit. This not only regulates satiation-appetite balance, but it helps you savor the flavor and appreciate your loved ones.

66

The things we **rush through in life**, just to get them over with, are things

we don't value.

In our crazy, hurried lives we often **rush through mealtime**, giving kids the subtle but distinct **message** that **we don't value it.**

99

1.5 FROM DIETING TO EATING DISORDERS

As a Brave Parent, it's crucial to be aware of warning signs that stray from healthy eating. Eating disorders describe illnesses that are characterized by irregular eating habits and severe distress or concern about body weight or shape. These may include inadequate or excessive food intake that can damage a child's well-being.

Eating pathologies such as anorexia and bulimia are both ways to control food. Anorexia affects girls more than boys, but boys represent one in every four children diagnosed with anorexia. Adolescent eating disorders stats show 2.7% of US teens (ages thirteen to eighteen) have an eating disorder. These years can also be an overlayed time of intense emotions, confusion, and stress for our kiddos. According to the 2009 Youth Risk Behavior Survey, 33% of adolescent girls believe they are overweight, and 56% are attempting to lose weight. And now, some teenagers are so fixated on "clean eating" that they've created a new category of anorexia.

How does it happen that we slip from normal eating patterns that fulfill our innate energy needs of the day to patterns of extreme control, frustration, body image distortion, and shame?

The day I first heard Professor Esther Parks lecturing my dental colleagues on signs of eating disorders, I felt like I went to the mountain and Moses delivered the tablets! I not only learned the telltale signs among my patients but took the blinders off about my own tendencies.

She openly addressed our diet-crazed culture. Just three days before that, I'd united with my dental team to begin the cabbage soup diet—one of many diets we had "fun" trying out together.

Dr. Parks reminded my colleagues that we all start out as healthy eaters. Then we become unhappy with our image and try an occasional diet, a controllable plan with a claim to help us lose weight. Today, I see no more fervency in my patients than in the first phase of a new diet. They are full of hope that *this* shiny new plan will finally give them the happiness they seek.

Most diets, while you're sticking to them, are initially successful, which is what makes them so alluring. But we subtly cross the line to *eating pathology* when we become a *chronic dieter*.

If you think we were chronically diet-crazed in the 1990s, take a look now. Overweight and unhealthy as ever before, our population is obsessed with losing weight. The diet industry collects upward of $78 billion a year.

My patients often seek my opinion on what diet is better: keto, paleo, vegan, or something else? I tell them, "They all work. And then they all let you down." Unless you can adopt a healthy relationship to food, to grow better preferences as a lifestyle habit rather than a diet plan, they won't work. I just love the quote by the non-diet health coach, Krista Murias: "Dieting steals your power to make your own decisions for your body. And then blames you when you fail."

Chronic cyclical dieters often have heightened negative emotions associated with food. Adopting rigid eating rules disconnects you from your physical and emotional health.

The guilt and shame from not being able to stick to your diet is what derails you. Furthermore, the diet culture has disparaged almost every food and food group from fat, eggs, bananas, dairy, lectins, gluten, grains, and meat.

If you are a chronic dieter and your child sees this, do them a favor and stop! (And by the way, they see *everything*.)

Many of us also engage in stress eating, reaching for a favorite "comfort food" to help manage anxiety. (Notice that comfort foods are rarely healthy foods.) If you see this pattern in you or your child, try to identify what is causing the emotional trigger for stress eating and address that, perhaps with a skilled therapist.

Equally prevalent are specific food addictions—especially to foods that contain sugar, fat, and/or salt. Food addiction is tricky because unlike alcohol, tobacco, and illicit drugs, no treatment method includes eliminating eating. We need food to survive! Children experience food addictions also. If you notice your child engaging in binging, craving, purging, or experiencing withdrawal symptoms from certain foods, let it serve as a red flag.

The goal is to develop good relationships with food, along with our children. Here's what it looks like: I *prefer* real food. I enjoy it, and it's satisfying. I'm aware of my hunger (and it's *real*, not manipulated by added sugar). The energy-rich foods I consume vary, based on my appetite. I don't need to worry about portion control. I don't need to diet to achieve or maintain a healthy weight.

To get there, start with the food pillars (above) and see how it changes your family dynamics, happiness, and health.

A word of warning: if you're watching your child struggle with pathologic eating, take it seriously as these disorders can be deadly. While we stand by hoping the condition will resolve itself, the diet culture is fueling disordered eating, so the odds are completely stacked against you. Seek help from a health professional who specializes in eating disorders. And remember: establishing a healthy relationship with food is never a sprint. It's a marathon ... and it's lifelong.

CONCLUSION

You are what you eat. You've heard this before but now I hope you really believe it. Your cells are screaming for the right nutrients—the building blocks for recovery and optimal health.

A serving of commercial, sugared-up yogurt and a juice box are not the answer. Nor is bargaining with kids for a "treat"—a bag of hot Cheetos, a blue Gatorade, Honey Nut Cheerios, or Reese's Peanut Butter Cups. I hope now you see that your child's body recognizes these as the exact opposite of treats. When it comes to metabolic health, these are truly evils.

As with so much in parenting, we each get a short window of opportunity to influence a child for a lifetime. This is yours. It's time to take your fridge, freezer, and pantry by storm. Own them. Don't let your kids dictate how you fill them, what you will offer. Your child's health and happiness depend on your day-to-day conversations and grocery store decisions.

Repeat your Brave Parent mantra as often as necessary: "My job is to provide healthy and appetizing foods for our children. Their job is to eat them when they're hungry.

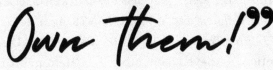

66 As with so much in parenting, we each get a short window of opportunity to **influence** a child for a lifetime. This is yours. It's time to take your fridge, freezer, and pantry by storm.

Own Them! **99**

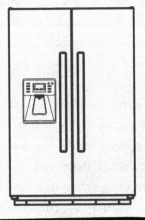

CHAPTER 1 REFERENCES

Ahima, R. S., & Antwi, D. A. (2008, December). *Brain regulation of appetite and satiety*. Endocrinology and metabolism clinics of North America. Retrieved September 22, 2021, from https://www.ncbi.nlm.nih.gov/pmc/articles/PMC2710609/.

Bale, B., Doneen, A., & Cool, L. C. (2014). *Beat the heart attack gene: The revolutionary plan to prevent heart disease, stroke, and diabetes.* Wiley.

CDC. (2017, November 16). *Only 1 in 10 adults get enough fruits or vegetables*. Centers for Disease Control and Prevention. Retrieved September 24, 2021, from https://www.cdc.gov/media/releases/2017/p1116-fruit-vegetable-consumption.html.

Centers for Disease Control and Prevention. (2021, February 8). *Products - HEALTH E stats - prevalence of Overweight, obesity, and severe obesity among children and ADOLESCENTS Aged 2–19 Years: United States, 1963–1965 Through 2017–2018.* Centers for Disease Control and Prevention. Retrieved September 9, 2021, from https://www.cdc.gov/nchs/data/hestat/obesity-child-17-18/obesity-child.htm.

FAD diets explained. American Association of Clinical Endocrinology. (n.d.). Retrieved September 20, 2021, from https://www.aace.com/disease-and-conditions/nutrition-and-obesity/fad-diets-explained.

Hébert, J. R., Shivappa, N., Wirth, M. D., Hussey, J. R., & Hurley, T. G. (2019, March 1). *Perspective: The dietary inflammatory index (dii)- lessons learned, improvements made, and future directions.* Advances in nutrition (Bethesda, Md.). Retrieved September 22, 2021, from https://www.ncbi.nlm.nih.gov/pmc/articles/PMC6416047/.

Justo, P. D. (2015, February 2). *The dirty truth about Doritos: What you're really eating on Super Bowl Sunday*. Salon. Retrieved September 22, 2021, from https://www.salon.com/2015/02/01/the_dirty_truth_about_doritos_what_youre_really_eating_on_super_bowl_sunday/.

Keller, A., & Della Torre, S. B. (2015, August). *Sugar-sweetened beverages and obesity among children and adolescents: A review of systematic literature reviews.* Childhood obesity (Print). Retrieved September 22, 2021, from https://www.ncbi.nlm.nih.gov/pmc/articles/PMC4529053/.

Lattimer, J. M., & Haub, M. D. (2010, December). *Effects of dietary fiber and its components on Metabolic Health.* Nutrients. Retrieved September 24, 2021, from https://www.ncbi.nlm.nih.gov/pmc/articles/PMC3257631/.

Lustig, R. H. (2014). *Fat chance: Beating the odds against sugar, processed food, obesity, and disease.* Plume.

Lustig, R. H. (2021). *Metabolical: The lure and the lies of processed food, nutrition, and Modern Medicine.* HarperWave, an imprint of HarperCollinsPublishers.

Mayo clinic staff. (2021, July 23). *Mediterranean diet for heart health.* Mayo Clinic. Retrieved September 22, 2021, from https://www.mayoclinic.org/healthy-lifestyle/nutrition-and-healthy-eating/in-depth/mediterranean-diet/art-20047801.

Moller, D. E., & Author Affiliations From the Charles A. Dana Research Institute and Harvard—Thorndike Laboratory of Beth Israel Hospital; the Department of Medicine. (1992, February 27). *Insulin resistance - mechanisms, syndromes, and implications: Nejm.* New England Journal of Medicine. Retrieved September 22, 2021, from https://www.nejm.org/doi/10.1056/NEJM199109263251307.

Moynihan, P. (2016, January 15). *Sugars and dental caries: Evidence for setting a recommended threshold for intake.* Advances in nutrition (Bethesda, Md.). Retrieved September 22, 2021, from https://www.ncbi.nlm.nih.gov/pmc/articles/PMC4717883/.

NIAID. (2014). *Immune Cells.* National Institute of Allergy and Infectious Diseases. Retrieved September 22, 2021, from https://www.niaid.nih.gov/research/immune-cells.

NIMH. (n.d.). *NIMH " eating disorders.* National Institute of Mental Health. Retrieved September 24, 2021, from https://www.nimh.nih.gov/health/statistics/eating-disorders.

Pollan, M. (2009). *Food Rules: An Eater's Manual.* Penguin Books.

Popkin, B. M., Adair, L. S., & Ng, S. W. (2012, January). *Global nutrition transition and the pandemic of obesity in developing countries.* Nutrition reviews. Retrieved September 22, 2021, from https://www.ncbi.nlm.nih.gov/pmc/articles/PMC3257829/.

Rippe, J. M., & Angelopoulos, T. J. (2016, November 4). *Relationship between added sugars consumption and chronic disease risk factors: Current understanding.* Nutrients. Retrieved September 22, 2021, from https://www.ncbi.nlm.nih.gov/pmc/articles/PMC5133084/.

Weiner, J. (2021, May 5). *The weight-loss industry is coming for our post-lockdown bodies.* The New York Times. Retrieved September 24, 2021, from https://www.nytimes.com/2021/05/05/opinion/culture/dieting-covid-weight-loss.html.

WHO. (2015). *Cancer: Carcinogenicity of the consumption of red meat and processed meat.* World Health Organization. Retrieved September 23, 2021, from https://www.who.int/news-room/q-a-detail/cancer-carcinogenicity-of-the-consumption-of-red-meat-and-processed-meat.

CHAPTER TWO

drink

BUBBLE, FIZZ, GUZZLE, GULP: WHAT IS THIS
STUFF ANYWAY?

INTRODUCTION

As I sit on my porch this morning, drinking my daily organic chai tea with a dash of whole cow's milk, I wonder ... what's really in my tea? I know it's black tea with a bunch of spices, but were all those spices *really* grown organically? I doubt it. And was the cow who gave that milk *really* grass-fed and antibiotic-free? Then there's the caffeine question. With 40 mg of caffeine per cup, (about one-third that of coffee), would it be better still for me to buy the decaffeinated version? What processing does the manufacturer have to do to remove the caffeine from the tea leaves?

All these questions that I ordinarily don't ponder because ... well, because ... I LOVE IT! There is something about the taste, the aroma, and the warmth. And *that*, my friends, is the criteria most of us use to choose our habitual drink-of-choice. The trouble is, many of our drinking habits are killing us, and we don't even know it.

Americans now consume nearly one hundred pounds of sugar per person each year. Nearly half of that comes from fruit drinks, sodas, and sports and energy drinks. Together such drinks are the top source of calories in the American diet—and the excessive sugar leads right to obesity, diabetes, cardiovascular disease, cancer, and depression.

It's worse now than ever. Since 1970, Americans' consumption of sugar-sweetened soda has *doubled* to an average of forty gallons a year per person—about two eight-ounce cans every day. And although soda consumption dropped to thirty-two gallons a year per person by 2011, we've more than made up for it with a spike in the consumption of sports drinks, vitamin water, energy drinks, and sweet teas, adding up to fourteen gallons a person per year. Summing it all up, we're averaging forty-five gallons a year now ... *per person*!

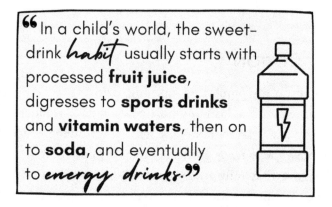

> " In a child's world, the sweet-drink *habit* usually starts with processed **fruit juice**, digresses to **sports drinks** and **vitamin waters**, then on to **soda**, and eventually to *energy drinks*. "

In a child's world, the sweet-drink habit usually starts with processed fruit juice, digresses to sports drinks and vitamin waters, then on to soda, and eventually to energy drinks. I'm here to tell you —they're all terrible for them! C'mon Brave Parents, we know this. So why do we still keep *any of it* in the fridge? I'm not here to inflict guilt, but to help you figure this out, once and for all.

Next, the question I frequently get from parents is, "What about sugar-free?" *Sugar-free* is an umbrella term used for all nonnutritive sweeteners (NNSs). Are any of these drinks better for us? Let me try to demystify that shortly.

Then, how about milk? Is dairy really inflammatory? Is almond milk better? Does soy milk speed up puberty? Is oat milk, which is low in fat and protein, okay for my toddler?

I also want to address a sensitive subject: caffeine. Sensitive because it treads on your own (probable) caffeine addiction. Let's face it. We are a caffeine-addicted culture, and our children are little addicts-in-training. How much caffeine is too much for kids? What are the risks and benefits? And at what age is it actually safe?

Finally, there's water. About 60% of our body is made up of it, and half of us don't get enough. But to drink it straight-up is so BORING—especially against the backdrop of the unending beverage aisle in every grocery and convenient store across America. Plus, we don't even trust our tap water anymore. (As if a bright blue bottle of sugar-free Powerade is better for them. How do you spell "chemical shitstorm"?)

So, we wonder ... is bottled water better than tap? If so, *which* bottled water? And is there any harm in drinking from single-use plastic containers—aside from the devastating impact it's having on the environment we're bestowing upon our kids?

Is it best to filter our water? If so, what about fluoride (which we talk about in chapter 7 Chew and Smile)? Is that filtered too?

Full disclosure: I don't have all the answers. I can hardly keep up with the food and beverage manufacturers' new "innovations," so I'm googling and PubMed searching as I go.

I just finished my chai, and I'm crossing my fingers as I chug a glass of well water on this beautiful Michigan morning.

2.1 JUICE FOR KIDS

In good conscience, I could start and end this subject with a simple sentence: Just say no! But I guess I owe you an explanation or two. Here are twenty.

Giving your kids juice of any kind is a precursor for trouble. They love the sweet taste. It's such a treat. And we justify it by reassuring ourselves it's "100% juice, with no added sugar." But with every sip, we're training their brains to have a *preference* for something cold and sweet to quench their thirst. That will come back to bite them ... and you. If you don't want to argue with your teenager about the quantity of sports drinks or sodas they are drinking at their friends' homes after school, get your toddler hooked on water.

I'm surprised that many pediatricians are still recommending juice for infants as a preventive measure for constipation, since the American Academy of Pediatrics (AAP) clearly endorses that fruit juice *not* be given to children younger than age one. Though in fairness, I usually hear only one side of the story. I hear about the docs' juice recommendations secondhand from an angry and frustrated parent, while I'm tasked with filling a mouthful of cavities on their two- or three-year-old. Partly to blame might be an un-Brave Parent who succumbs to their kiddo's nagging demands after they're hooked.

So, what are the recommendations for painful constipation? There are three particular juices that help: prune, apple, and pear. It seems juice can be given safely once babies are four months old but should be limited to two to three ounces of 100% fruit juice per day. You can give up to six ounces of fruit juice per day to infants eight to twelve months old. For any age, fruit juice is not recommended for daily consumption for more than a week or two. Plus, to help protect their precious teeth, don't give it to them within an hour of bedtime.

It might go without saying, but I'll say it anyway: I don't recommend buying juice that has added sugar ... ever! I'm not just talking about Capri Sun and Hawaiian Punch; this includes cranberry and cran-apple juice. (By the way, have you ever eaten a cranberry without the sugar? It's practically inedible.)

One of the problems with fruit juice is it's missing most of the benefits of the *whole* fruit. Gone is the *fiber* (our kids' *number one nutrient deficiency*). Gone are most of our plant-based micronutrients (called phytonutrients), the building blocks of cell health. Here to stay is the sugar water. Juice has lots of the worst kind of sugar too

—*fructose* which is processed in the liver. Without the fiber to slow absorption and mitigate the insulin release, we are setting kids up for weight gain and other serious metabolic challenges such as insulin resistance and nonalcoholic fatty liver disease. (To learn more, revisit chapter 1 Eat and chapter 3 Digest.)

Scientific data also suggests that liquid calories fail to trigger the same hunger satisfaction in the brain that solid foods do. That implicates regular consumption of 100% fruit juices in the obesity epidemic—even those with added fiber.

If all that's not enough, please note that drinking near-empty juice calories will displace your kiddo's appetite for other nutrient-rich foods. It's true. We've been aware for decades that too much fruit juice consumption is linked to micronutrient malnutrition (MM). With MM, a child may not look underweight, but their inadequate intake of vitamins and minerals interrupts the body's ability to produce enzymes, hormones, and other essential elements for proper growth and development. In 2021 the World Health Organization (WHO) stated that at least *half* of all children under five, worldwide, suffer from it.

Enough about juice. It's time to repeat that simple sentence: Just say NO.

2.2 SODA

Now that you know how vehement I am about leaving juice in the grocery store, I'm sure you can guess how much I despise the entire soda industry—pocketing their profits on the backs of our declining health. I wish it were illegal! But since it's not, you as a Brave Parent can make it illegal in your own house—and not just for your kiddos, for the adults too. As much as you might want to label these as "off-limits adult beverages," kids yearn for a sip if they see it in your hands. We chide them to "Do as I say, not as I do." but you know that's just plain opposite what we see over time.

One of the problems with **fruit juice** is it's missing most of the benefits of the *whole fruit.* Gone is the **fiber** (our kids' number one nutrient deficiency).

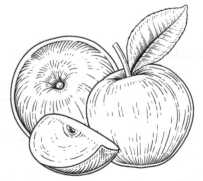

Gone are most of our **plant-based micronutrients** (called phytonutrients), the building blocks of **cell health**. Here to stay is the sugar water.

Many families who choose not to keep soda in the house allow kids to order it whenever they eat out, as sort of a "special treat." Remember the #2 Food Pillar in chapter 1 Eat? It says, "Don't use food as a reward or punishment." That goes for drinks too. Does it make any sense that we would elevate to "treat" status a substance as inherently bad for your child's health as soda? Nope!

So why do I think it's so bad for you? I simply can't count the ways. Beyond all the chemical flavorings and colorings, caffeine, and its inherent acidity, soda is laden with high-fructose corn syrup (HFCS), one of the most dangerous threats on the planet to our children's health, and that's not about to change any time soon.

With corn subsidized by the government, cheap corn turned into cheap corn-sweetener, and HFCS took over the soda industry. As people learned of its dangers, the industry designed several aliases (such as glucose-fructose, maize syrup, high-fructose maize syrup, isoglucose, glucose isolate, and corn syrup) in order to obscure your ability to recognize HFCS on the ingredient list.

The plot thickens. During a handful of decades, average serving sizes swelled from 7 oz in the 1950s to the "medium-sized" 32 oz drink at your favorite fast-food joint. It's not unusual for my soda-drinking patients to suck down five or six 20-ounce screw-top bottles throughout each and every day. These, by the way, are very sick patients with very sick teeth. Tooth decay is just a smoke signal. They also suffer from every lifestyle-related disease on our radar, and they usually don't understand why.

Teens and adults don't wake up one day and decide to guzzle a gallon of soda. And they usually can't quit overnight either. A cold-turkey end to these caffeine and sugar addictions can cause serious detox symptoms at any age, and they'll do just about anything to avoid that. But not just kids and teens, adults too!

I remember visiting my brother-in-law in the hospital the day after his emergency quadruple bypass surgery. I called ahead to ask if there was anything I could possibly bring to comfort this sweet man, who'd just had his chest cracked open following a heart attack. My sister reported, "He'd really like a cold Mountain Dew. They don't have it here in the hospital." (Are you kidding me??) The tragic irony was not lost on me.

2.3 SPORTS DRINKS

Skipping the soda and reaching for popular sports drinks may seem like a healthy choice, but they're not much better than soda when it comes to sugar. A 32 oz sports drink contains between 56 g and 76 g of sugar—about fourteen to nineteen teaspoons. That's about four to five times more sugar than your child should be consuming ... for the entire day!

That's not just my opinion. I'm basing that on the WHO sugar consumption guidelines: 5% of a person's total energy intake. That calculates to four teaspoons a day (or 16 g) for four- to eight-year-olds, based on a daily average calorie intake of 1300. It jumps to five teaspoons for nine- to thirteen-year-olds, who average 1700 calories a day.

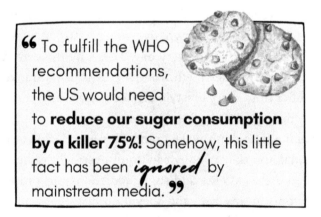

66 To fulfill the WHO recommendations, the US would need to **reduce our sugar consumption by a killer 75%!** Somehow, this little fact has been *ignored* by mainstream media. **99**

By the way, to fulfill the WHO recommendations, the US would need to reduce our sugar consumption by a killer 75%! Somehow this little fact has been ignored by mainstream media.

So, I just got a call from Meghan, one of my team members, who is standing on the sidelines at her daughter's travel softball tournament.

She said, "It's so hard to see what the parents have packed for their kids to eat and drink. I mean, these are competitive athletes, and they're living on hot Cheetos and bright blue Gatorade. It's just not right! The other parents are shocked that my kids drink *only* water. And they were practically mystified when they saw Austynn eating an avocado right out of the shell, with a spoon. Someone had the guts to ask her, 'What *is* that?'"

Meghan would be the first to tell you that, as a Brave-Parent-in-Training, she doesn't always get it right. But she has enough of the pieces in place that her kids are already seen as weirdos—and, lucky for them, they're assured a healthier future.

Do you ever wonder how sports drinks got the reputation as performance-enhancing health drinks? The same Gatorade that sits in the sideline's coolers today is now fifty-six years old. But *is* it the same? Not even close.

I'll never forget my first taste of Gatorade as a little kid. I had to spit it out! It tasted *nasty*—like a salty chemical spill. The original drink was developed by Drs. Robert Cade and Dana Shires in response to the exhaustion and dehydration that college football players suffered in the hot Florida sun. It was reported that some of the Florida Gators would lose fifteen pounds during a three-hour game, and Dr. Cade, a kidney specialist, sought a way to boost their electrolyte-rich plasma (the fluid part of the blood) during play.

The electrolytes Cade focused on were sodium and potassium, so he added sodium citrate and monopotassium to the mix. But the original amount of lemon-lime flavoring and fructose were not enough to overpower the awful taste of this stuff, and I wasn't the only one to spit it out. Players complained it tasted like a cross between urine and the toilet bowl cleaner itself. They had to add an artificial sweetener, much sweeter than sugar, just to get them to drink it.

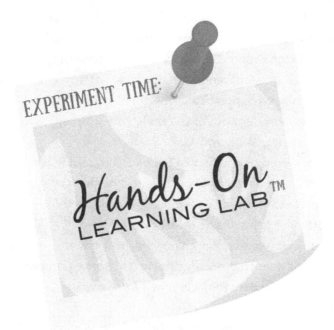

EXPERIMENT TIME:

Hands-On™
LEARNING LAB

This experiment will help your child **visualize the amount of sugar** in their favorite sweet drink.

Here's what you'll need:

- Sugar
- Teaspoon
- Calculator
- Funnel
- Clear Empty Bottle
- Child's Favorite Sweet Drink

Here's what you'll do:

With a teaspoon and a bowl of sugar, funnel in the amount of sugar indicated on the label. **A spoonful of sugar is equivalent to 4g.**

For example, if you have a 28oz bottle of Powerade Mountain Berry Blast in your hand, you will see the top two ingredients are water and sugar. **How much sugar?** The label says 21g. But now look at the serving size, 12oz.

There are about two and a half servings in that bottle, or 52g in the whole container. Assuming your kiddo is not sharing his bottle of Powerade with one and a half of his or her closest friends, **that 52g of sugar contains thirteen teaspoons of sugar!** Spoon it out into a heap and watch their eyes bug out in shock!

When Gatorade was sold to Quaker Oats in 1983, Fruit Punch Gatorade made its debut. Now it's owned by PepsiCo, and, no joke, it's their fourth largest brand. They dumped in a bunch more HFCS (or alternatively artificial sweeteners which we'll cover in a minute), and now it's not what Cade set out to do at all. He was clearly trying to help his athletes ... and that's plainly not happening.

As you know, Gatorade comes in all kinds of iridescent colors and a variety of sizes. It competes with Coca-Cola's Powerade and Vitaminwater brands, as well as several others that vie for a higher position in the still-soaring sports drink market.

Vitaminwater has the unearned perception of a healthier choice. Coca-Cola's marketing campaign assigned descriptors like *focus, endurance, refresh*, and *essential*. It's true, it contains vitamins, just as all our candied-up breakfast cereals do. But it has virtually the same whopping dose of sugar (32 g per 20 oz) as Gatorade and Powerade (35 g). Even for your teen athletes, a single bottle of Vitaminwater is more than 100% of the sugar intake they can healthily consume—*for the entire day*! You heard that right.

Not so incidentally, the American Heart Association (AHA) issued the exact same recommendation as the WHO, that your teenager have no more than six teaspoons (or 25 g) of added sugar per day. (We'll get to the sugar-free varieties in a minute.)

These sugar guidelines might sound strict, but I assure you they're not. Remember that one in five US kids is obese, and almost *half* are overweight.

I implore you, Brave Parents, to join efforts with the WHO, that has a particular focus on stabilizing (and eventually preventing) unhealthy weight gain and dental caries. And also with the AHA in their determination to reduce the threat of all noncommunicable diseases (NCDs) in your children, who will, in the blink of an eye, be adults.

By now you probably can't wait to hear me indict energy drinks. Yes, I find them the scourge of the earth. But hang tight till we get there ... after we talk about diet drinks and coffee.

2.4 SUGAR-FREE ANYONE?

"Sugar" is an umbrella term for caloric sweeteners: high-fructose corn syrup, cane sugar, honey, beet sugar, fruit juice concentrates, maple syrup, agave, and the list goes on. (There are now fifty-six common names for sugar.)

Likewise, "sugar-free" is the umbrella term for noncaloric sweeteners. The scientific term is *nonnutritive sweeteners* (NNSs), and these include sucralose (Splenda), aspartame (NutraSweet and Equal), acesulfame-K (Sweet One), neotame (Newtame), and saccharin (Sweet'N Low). There are now seventy-six names for NNSs.

Sucralose is the world's most commonly used NNS, and it's about 600 times more potent as a sweetener than table sugar. That's typical of the NNSs—they range from about 200 to 700 times more sweetness per volume. Because we have to use so little to make it sickly sweet, it earns the "zero calories" claim.

While attending an oral systemic health conference, I signed up for a fascinating workshop called "How Sweet It Is," sponsored by one of the NNS manufacturers. In the room were trays and trays of little white paper cups, filled with various clear liquids. Throughout the lecture, we proceeded to taste-test each of the most ubiquitous artificial sweeteners on the market.

Similar to a wine-tasting experience (except I actually enjoy the taste of wine), we were asked to describe the experience of each one —recording its relative sweetness, palatability, length of time it lingered, aftertaste, etc. That day I learned *how* and *why* the manufacturers assign particular sweeteners to various sugar-free gums, candies, yogurts, salad dressings, and sweet drinks—all in an effort to mimic the real deal. One of the presenters emphasized that food scientists are always working to make our food more palatable, for a more enjoyable eating experience.

Then one lone soul in back of the room raised her hand. A young dentist from California respectfully asked, *"Why* are we training people to enjoy the taste of all these bizarre chemicals? This can't be healthy for us, can it? I mean, why not just retrain people to enjoy the taste of *real* food?" The speaker was stunned for a moment, preparing a reply, when I began to applaud. Soon there was an entire percussion section of supporters, and the room vibrated with energy over the controversy. I did feel a little sorry for the presenter, whose pitch had been hijacked.

I remember feeling grateful for that brave disruptor. She reminded us just how *uncommon* is common sense these days and that pumping our food and beverage supply full of artificial sweeteners doesn't make sense at all. But before you conclude that for yourself, let's look at the literature.

There are numerous evidence gaps about the health and safety of NNSs. Perhaps the most researched NNS in the US is aspartame, with over one hundred studies behind it. It has been approved by the Food and Drug Administration (FDA) since 1981, and its safety as an ingested chemical is not so much in question. Keep in mind the FDA and most published studies (especially industry-funded ones) endorse the safety of *all* these NNSs, or they wouldn't be on the market.

It's not the toxicity of artificial sweeteners, but the *metabolic effects* on the body we are most dubious about today.

We have data from several epidemiological studies that consumption of NNSs, mainly in diet sodas, is associated with increased risk of developing obesity, type 2 diabetes, and metabolic syndrome (a large waist, increased blood pressure, high triglyceride level, risky blood cholesterol ratio, and elevated fasting blood sugar).

I don't know about you, but I don't want my kiddos to have *any* of those! (Actually, I *do* know about you because you're on my Brave Parent team!)

If you're curious why these NNSs are labeled as "metabolically inactive" but seem to promote what we call *metabolic dysregulation*, there are currently three potential mechanisms: (1) NNSs interfere with our learned responses that contribute to our glucose-insulin control, (2) NNSs interfere with our gut microbiome and stimulate glucose intolerance, and (3) NNSs interact with the sweet taste receptors that are distributed throughout our digestive tract. They, too, play a role in glucose absorption and insulin secretion.

Before I leave the subject of NNSs, I want to mention one in particular that has been highly therapeutic for my cavity-prone patients. *Xylitol* (in the polyol family) is a naturally found sweetener, extracted from the bark of the birchwood tree. In the mouth, it has the opposite effect on the oral bacteria that cause cavities. (See section 7.4 on Caries Disease in chapter 7 Chew and Smile.) While the cavity bugs normally *eat* sugar and *pee* acid on your teeth, eating xylitol causes these bugs to become *constipated*, quelling the acid bath.

Finland was way ahead of the US in using xylitol to help control caries disease, and with huge success. Their dental health promotion efforts began in 1991 with the use of xylitol chewing gum and was super effective in dropping their cavity rates. Currently, more than half of all Finnish schoolchildren benefit from it.

Not so incidentally, xylitol is reported not to contribute to metabolic dysregulation and early studies show it may even be beneficial in reducing the progression of insulin resistance to type 2 diabetes

Personally, I'm quick to recommend xylitol candy and gum to my cavity-prone, dry-mouth *adult* patients, including elderly and cancer patients. I'm more hesitant to prescribe it for children if they have dogs at home. Xylitol is extremely toxic to dogs. Even small amounts of xylitol can cause low blood sugar, seizures, liver failure, or even death in dogs, so it has to be stored up and out of reach. Kids are haphazard and if they have a pup, they need help from parents to regulate that. Call me a softy on this subject. It's not that I love kids' dogs more than their teeth, but you can bet *they* do.

Beyond dentistry, xylitol studies are continually bringing forward good evidence for its uses in reducing inflammation of mucous and sinus membranes, relieving constipation, improving bone mineral density, and fortifying the gut microbiome.

Keep your eye on the horizon for erythritol, another polyol. New studies reveal that erythritol might work even better to reduce dental plaque acids and the bugs that cause them, also without the metabolic dysregulation we see in the other NNSs.

2.5 HOW ABOUT COW'S MILK?

Let's start with the 2018 study that found chocolate milk was better than commercial sports drinks for boosting recovery after strenuous exercise. The athletes in the chocolate milk group apparently exercised intensely without tiring for six minutes longer than the sports drink group did.

It's true that milk has some electrolytes, and chocolate syrup has some added carbs, but what's also true is that most kids don't need the 200-ish replacement calories or the seventeen grams of added sugar ... *per one-cup serving.* They're hardly exercising like the Florida Gators, all-out for three to five hours on a blazing hot day.

Cow's milk has garnered a tough rap sheet during the last decade. Dairy, in general, has been somewhat demonized as a trigger for systemic inflammation and mucous production. That's especially true for lactose-sensitive or casein-allergic kids. The consensus is that around 80% of children with a cow's milk allergy will outgrow it by the time they're three to five years old.

There doesn't seem to be conclusive evidence supporting increased mucous production in kids who don't have dairy sensitivity, but be quick to initiate a dairy-free "holiday" if you suspect this might be helpful. You'll know if milk was a contributing factor within a couple weeks.

Weighing the pros and cons among the collective publications, I still find cow's milk beneficial for kids as long as they are consuming it in moderation. You don't want your child filling up on milk and missing the nutrient-dense vegetables and fruits their bodies crave most.

66

~~Chocolate~~ Milk

"It's true that milk has some electrolytes, and chocolate syrup has some added carbs, but what's also true is that most kids *don't need* the 200-ish replacement calories or the **seventeen grams of added sugar** ... per one-cup serving."

99

Cow's milk is a natural source of protein, calcium, potassium, and vitamin B_{12}. And it's *fortified* with vitamin D (meaning that it's added to the cow's milk during processing). Vitamin D is on every researcher's "top five" list of nutrient deficiencies in the US.

Cow's milk is considered safe to give children after they're a year old, but a child who is one or two years old should only drink *whole* milk. This is because the fat is essential for your child's developing brain.

I probably don't need to remind you not to give your little one unpasteurized milk. But I might need to remind you to buy only milk from cows that are treated humanely (grass-fed, antibiotic-free, and hormone-free). Look for milk that's labeled *Certified Humane* to make sure the cows were not dosed with genetically engineered hormones (such as rBGH or rBST) to increase milk production.

2.6 NUT MILK, SOY MILK, OAT MILK, AND BEYOND ...

There are several safe and somewhat healthful milks on the market today. Don't ask me what it looks like to "milk" an almond, a soybean, or the groat of an oat (oof!) ... but they all have merits.

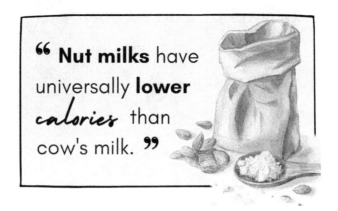

> **Nut milks** have universally **lower** *calories* than cow's milk.

Though none of these milks offer the protein content of traditional dairy, they bring plenty of nutrition of their own. Ounce for ounce, nut milks have universally lower calories than cow's milk, and many of them have at least as much (or more) calcium and vitamin D. Almond milk is the lowest in calories—as long as you don't buy an added-sugar variety. Beware of the vanilla or other flavored milks or creamers. If it sounds at all un-plain, check the label for added sugar just to be sure. While you're at it, notice the other chemical additives: salt, flavors, gums, emulsifiers, and other binding agents.

If you want to avoid all that, you should know that grain and nut milks (from oats, almonds, macadamia, hazelnuts, and cashews) are easy to make at home. All you need is a good blender (or grinder) and a strainer bag. Buy the nut milk bags online, then search that process on Google or YouTube.

But let's face it. Amidst the commotion of other Brave-Parent-energy-sucking stuff, most of us don't have the time *or* the interest in milking nuts. Seriously though, I challenge you to try it *once* just to see how easy it is. By the way, if you have school-age kiddos, you can teach them how to do it and then put them in charge.

2.7 WAKE-UP CALL ON CAFFEINE

We're clearly a caffeine-obsessed culture. And we're so good at training our kids to be addicted that by the time they advance to college age, 93% of them drink this drug *daily*. That's because 73% of us buy and serve our five- to twelve-year-olds caffeine in our homes. (Well, at least I assume that's where they get it, since this age group doesn't drive or shop, and 73% of them slug it down *daily*.) These stats confound me, considering the American Academy of Pediatrics (among other kid authorities) say children *under the age of twelve should avoid caffeine* altogether.

In 2013 I complained to a fourteen-year-old patient that Mountain Dew had just launched a juice-like breakfast drink. He chimed in, "Really? I thought Mountain Dew already *was* a breakfast drink! ... At least it is in *our* house."

Maybe that grosses you out because *you*, like me, wouldn't even think about drinking a substance that looks exactly like the antifreeze you put in your car. But you don't feel quite so terrified by the aroma of your morning coffee. If you're a coffee lover, do you remember your first sip? It was bitter and strange. You trained your brain to enjoy it because it promised to pep you up. And now you're showing your kids how it's done.

Once again, it's time to look at our own habits. After all, our kids surely do! I'm not trying to demonize a cup of coffee (and certainly not my organic chai tea, LOL), but I have concerns about our ever-growing reliance on this wildly compelling drug.

Caffeine is a white alkaloid powder, derived from coffee beans or tea leaves, and sprinkled into anything drinkable. But wait—is it a drug?

In 1958 caffeine was classified by the FDA as a *food additive* on the GRAS list (Generally Recognized as Safe). It *is* truly a drug, but its status was complicated by the fact that it occurs naturally in foods such as chocolate, coffee beans, and tea leaves. (Let me remind you that opioids are naturally found in the poppy plant, but that doesn't make them safe for everyday use.)

Caffeine has its merits. It is considered a mildly addictive, psychoactive drug. It will increase your alertness, especially if you only use it once in a while. Caffeine blocks the sleep hormone (adenosine) receptors in your brain to keep you from feeling sleepy.

When it's consumed regularly, in moderation (less than 400 mg per day), it shows some promising health benefits, such as reducing risk for type 2 diabetes (according to one study). Another study showed caffeine to improve athletic performance in sprints and endurance activities lasting up to two hours.

Caffeine is also associated with negative health consequences when you consume too much, including increased heart rate, palpitations, insomnia, anxiety, increased blood pressure, bladder instability, GI distress (diarrhea), and pregnancy complications.

But my biggest beef isn't with the caffeine itself—it's with what we add to it. What do these have in common: Starbucks caramel latte, Coffee mate French vanilla creamer, Coke, Pepsi, Red Bull, and Rockstar? It's SUGAR, the primary ingredient. (Oh, that again!) Remember that sugar underlies our epidemics of tooth decay, obesity, and type 2 diabetes, while the *acidity* of *all* these liquids promotes osteoporosis and kidney stones. I trust you don't want any of these conditions for your children as they grow into adulthood.

When it comes to caffeine, being brave means reducing or cutting your own consumption—perhaps leaving it in the grocery store altogether. If you choose to quit cold turkey or even do a hard reset, starting with a twenty-one-day "caffeine holiday," you might experience a few days of withdrawal symptoms. The most common complaint is headaches. Keep in mind that many over-the-counter headache remedies contain a bit of caffeine, which will help you during those first couple days.

> **66** Talk instead about how *unnecessary* **caffeine** is for a **healthy person** and **warn** your kids about the possible *dangers* of consuming too much. **99**

2.8 ENERGY DRINKS ARE ALL THE RAGE

The worst of all evil drinks are energy drinks like Red Bull, Mountain Dew Amp, and Rockstar Pure Zero. I can hardly believe that 42% of

US adults (ages thirty to forty-nine) are drinking this stuff. All I can say is ... if *you* are, stop it! Your kids are watching, and they certainty don't need your help with the advertising.

With brightly colored packaging and youthful advertisements, energy drink marketing efforts target children, tweens, and teens. I have to ask *why* this is legal when the American Academy of Pediatrics clearly states that children should not consume these products?

Because even more serious than caffeine addiction and withdrawal is *caffeine intoxication* from crazy amounts of consumption. Whereas a typical cup of coffee delivers a 90 mg jolt, energy drinks will dispense two or three times that in one 16 oz can.

Between 2007 and 2011, the number of US emergency department visits due to energy drink overdose doubled from 10,068 to 20,783. That's according to the US Substance Abuse and Mental Health Services Administration.

Caffeine overdose is highest among males in the eighteen- to twenty-four-year-old age group, and it's often associated with late-night partying. That's because energy shots are often pumped into designer cocktails, a pump or two at a time, at about 100 mg per shot.

A few years ago, during his junior year in college, my nephew told me about the latest cocktail of choice: Jägermeister, Red Bull, and—wait for it—Viagra! (That's *some* kind of party waiting to happen. Ugh!) You can see how hard it would be for them to regulate their caffeine consumption—especially when they're under the influence of booze, not to mention an erectile stimulant.

Alas, when a fellow partier begins to have seizures, someone calls an ambulance. By then, they've probably ignored the precursors which might include a case of the jitters, rapid heart rate, nausea, anxiety, heart arrhythmia, sweating, or vomiting. When death occurs, it's from cardiac arrest.

Incidentally, among this same young adult population, energy drinks are linked to increased substance abuse and risk-taking behaviors.

Do you see why I think energy drinks are wicked? And I'm not alone. The WHO also warns that "increased consumption of energy drinks may pose a serious danger to public health, especially among young people."

Enough already! You get it. And here, Brave Parents, is your call to action. Keep that stuff out of your own body, out of your house, and completely out of the realm of possibilities for your kiddos!

Talk instead about how *unnecessary* caffeine is for a healthy person and warn your kids about the possible dangers of consuming too much. For an energy boost, foster their habits of good nutrition, lots of high-quality sleep, and plenty of water.

> " For an *energy boost*, foster their habits of good **nutrition**, lots of high-quality **sleep**, and plenty of **water**. "

2.9 THAT LEAVES … WATER!

Now that I've single-handedly condemned every one of your and your kiddo's favorite drinks, you are probably feeling guilty and glum. (I'm truly sorry about that.)

What's left to drink, you ask. What do *you* think?

Water!

Yup, water. It helps your kiddo regulate body temperature, lubricate and cushion their joints, protect their spinal cord and other sensitive tissues, get rid of wastes through urination, perspiration, and bowel movements, and just plain feel better. In short, adequate hydration helps your body do what it needs to do every day.

I promise you this, Brave Parents: If you keep your fridge and cupboards clean, starting your kiddos on plain water and *whole fruits* rather than fruit juices, they will grow up to *prefer* water to sweet drinks.

2.10 HOW MUCH WATER SHOULD KIDS DRINK?

A good rule of thumb, and one easy to remember, is kids need one 8 oz glass of water per day, for each year of life. For example, a four-year-old should be drinking four glasses (or about 32 oz). After eight years old, the 64 oz recommendation maxes out and extends on into adulthood. I know we talked about the benefits of different milks, and if you choose to give your kiddo a glass of milk, you won't want to reduce their water to compensate.

"How much water?" is a much easier question to answer than "*What kind* of water?" should your kiddo drink?

2.11 WATER, WATER EVERYWHERE ... AND NOT A DROP TO DRINK!

That's how almost half of Americans feel about tap water. The 2014 Flint, Michigan, river water scandal tainted *all* our perceptions about the safety of the government-sanctioned water coming to our own kitchen sinks. That was such a sad story of racial injustice and bad decision-making when the city officials switched Flint's water supply from Detroit (city water) to the Flint River in order to save money. (The river was a former "unofficial" waste disposal site used by local businesses that flourished along its shores.)

Knowing there was inadequate testing, officials still ignored residents' complaints, and it resulted in significant health deterioration, including elevated blood *lead* levels in their children.

When the scandal blew up internationally, the United Nations responded, sponsoring a "World Water Day" celebration. They brought in twelve semitrailers stacked with pallets of free bottled water on the city's street corners, offering them to any city resident who could show an ID. The whole world breathed a sigh of relief when single-use bottles of water came to the rescue.

Now, Flint, Michigan has as good (or better) water quality as anyone else in my state, but its residents still don't trust it. Most of them still drink bottled water. (And maybe you do, too, as a result.) It's actually the political officials they still don't trust. And can you blame them?

Nine government officials were charged with willful neglect of their residents, though later the charges were mysteriously dropped. In my mind, these "leaders" did much more than hurt their residents. They shamefully eroded public confidence about the safety of tap water throughout *our entire country*.

Many people now perceive bottled water as the cleanest form of potable water without knowing anything about its origins. Keep in mind, when you buy bottled water, the source of the water is most likely unclear.

Those who prefer bottled water often claim they can even taste the difference. Truth is, that's all wrapped up with our mindset. In repeated blind taste tests, we fail to discern the difference.

Now let me give you another perspective on drinking water. The US Environmental Protection Agency (EPA) is responsible for the safety of 150,000 public water systems across the US that serve more than 300 million people. Conversely, the FDA is responsible for overseeing the countless brands of bottled water.

The EPA, through its Safe Drinking Water Act, has historically been even *more* stringent about tap water bacterial counts than was the FDA about bottled water, though now the bacteria safety of bottled water appears to have caught up.

Of course, the EPA guidelines for tap water are upheld at the treatment facility and do not extend once the distribution process has begun. Depending on your home's plumbing situation, the water could decrease in quality by the time it reaches your faucet. The same holds true for well water. Many health departments and private companies offer free water testing, and I encourage you to take advantage of that. Take the sample from your kitchen sink, the primary source of drinking and cooking water.

Then, if you identify a need for purifying your water, think about investing in a home filtration system, such as reverse osmosis. Filtration also removes chlorine or chloramine, the tap water disinfectants that have done their job and are no longer necessary.

As a dentist, I'm compelled to mention that reverse osmosis will filter out fluoride, too, so you'll need to seek a prescription supplement from your dentist to strengthen your kid's tooth enamel as it's forming. Incidentally, most bottled waters also lack fluoride. (See chapter 7 Chew and Smile for much more on fluoride.)

There are other health threats to consider regarding bottled water. Acidifying consumable liquids is the easiest way to keep bacterial counts down and extend their shelf life, since the liquids sit still in warehouses and stores. As such, bottled waters are all over the grid on their acidity. Many bottled waters have a pH of 4—1000 times more acidic than tap water. In fact, some of the most popular brands, offered by the biggest beverage manufacturers, are the most acidic—and they're not healthy as a go-to beverage.

Quick science lesson: The acid-base pH scale spans from 1 (like battery acid) to 14 (like Clorox bleach). The middle number, 7, is neutral; that's where our body (blood and saliva) like to be. Tap water is neutral also. The pH scale runs up and down from 7 with a *geometric progression*, meaning each number is a multiplier of ten. So, a pH of 6 is ten times more acidic than neutral. A pH of 5 is one hundred times more acidic, and so on. It's shocking to learn that our most popular sodas have a pH of 3—*10,000 times* more acidic than tap water ... or your body. It's terrible for your teeth, for starters.

When I see patients with yellowed, sensitive, lackluster teeth, I know they've suffered from *enamel erosion* (thinning of the enamel surface) from the acid. Getting curious, I usually discover they've been sipping on sodas, lemon water, or ... you guessed it ... *single-serving bottled water*. To buffer the acid attack, we release calcium from our teeth. That's what causes enamel erosion, and its likely leaching calcium out of our bones as well. Habitually drinking such acidic beverages is also linked to osteoporosis and kidney stones.

Next, you'll want to consider the substances used to make these single-use water bottles that pretend to be inert. They're nasty plastic polymers that allow chemicals to leach out, contaminating the water and thus your body. We worry *most* about the endocrine disruptors such as bisphenol A (BPA), which has been linked to breast cancer, endocrine dysfunctions in fetuses and children, obesity, and organ damage. But there are other plastic toxins too. I'm pretty sure it would only take one field trip to the factory sidelines to get a big whiff of these bottles hot off the production line for us to refuse them forever more!

High temperature storage enhances the chemical release, like when you leave a bottle of water in your hot car and return to it later. It's easy to grasp this, since most of us have banned plastic containers and plastic bags from our microwave. (I've also stopped storing leftovers in plastic containers.)

Thinner plastic bottles are more crinkle-able and are rumored to release more chemicals than the thicker ones. But it seems to me the thicker ones pose an even uglier environmental impact. On average it takes 450 years to degrade a single bottle!

So, let's talk seriously about the horrific environmental impact of single-use plastic, because you know, Brave Parents, we're setting our kids up for a world of hurt. We heap about four *billion* plastic water bottles a year into the US waste stream. That's *if* the bottle makes it into the landfill; many end up in the wilderness and water-ways, wreaking devastation on our wildlife.

Think about this: Plastic didn't even enter the public sphere until the 1950s, and now look at us. It's only been seventy years, and single-use plastic bottles have become a catastrophic contributor to ocean *and* land pollution. I am fantasizing about a massive Brave Parent movement that could stimulate this nonsense to stop!

Bottled water is also ridiculously expensive. Where tap water costs about three bucks per 1000 liters, bottled water costs three bucks for a *single* liter. That covers the cost to advertise, produce, distribute, store, discard, and *profit* from each of these components.

As it is, the entire life cycle of bottled water uses more than seventeen million barrels of oil a year to produce enough plastic water bottles to meet America's demand. In addition, we spend about $70 million a year in cleanup and maintenance of our landfills. This all seems like crazy business to me when we're already paying for safe tap water through our taxes!

2.12 WHAT ABOUT SPARKLING WATER?

Here's finally some good news for those of you who want a break in the monotony of plain water. The commonly held myth that the carbonation harms your teeth is just that ... a myth. There's simply no good scientific evidence that sparkling water hurts your teeth, your bones, *or* your body. Interestingly, a carbonated drink may even enhance digestion by improving swallowing ability and reducing constipation.

But before you head to the fridge (or the store), keep reading. Carbonated waters vary a bunch in their acidity. Flavored waters are mostly acidic—and with that added threat, you're back to the same issues we discussed a minute ago.

My favorite tasting fizzy water is grapefruit Bubly, but with a pH of 4, I know it's 1000 times more acid than tap water, so I drink it infrequently. I also like S.Pellegrino, which is unflavored, but has a pH of about 7, mirroring the neutrality of tap water and your saliva. My advice is to keep a small tablet of pH paper (a.k.a. litmus paper) on hand. It's super cheap and easy to find online. That way you can test everything you and your kids are drinking and treat them to a science lesson while you're at it.

My second piece of advice is to avoid single-use containers altogether by purchasing a SodaStream—a gadget that will allow you to add fun bubbles to your own tap water. The carbonation will not change the pH.

In some studies, carbonated water improved satiety, or the feeling of fullness, which can help people who constantly feel hungry. For the same reason, sparkling water may not be the best way to increase your water consumption.

CONCLUSION

Water. Drink it warm, drink it cold, drink it fizzy or still. But drink it!

And boycott single-use plastics!

Instead, have some fun shopping for and personalizing refillable water containers for everyone in your household. Make sure they're BPA-free, easy to clean, and appealing to use. Many companies are using safe, environmentally friendly materials such as stainless steel, recyclable bamboo, and food-grade silicone.

Hunter always enjoyed embellishing his with a unique collection of adventure stickers. If your kiddo carries a backpack, tuck it in or get a carabiner clip to hook it on the outside. Drinking from a personalized container makes it easy for everyone in your family to track their daily consumption.

As you're making significant changes in your household drinking habits, turn your water drinking into a fun challenge. Find creative ways to track intake and offer rewards. Include the adults too—that helps keep everyone accountable.

By the way, I didn't mention alcohol in this chapter because, well, it shouldn't pertain to kids, but while I'm concluding, let me challenge you. If you drink alcohol, drink in moderation and, by all means, drink responsibly. Never drink and drive. Be careful not to elevate your excitement about your latest designer cocktails.

Remember, you have kids in training, and all eyes are on you. If your alcohol consumption seems out of your control at times, or your parenting personality changes, or you become reliant on it for a daily numb-out, consider jumping on a Zoom AA meeting and living this day alcohol-free.

Together, as you change your household drinking habits, you'll all feel healthier—I promise. Look at it this way: by the time you eliminate the juice, soda, sports drinks, energy drinks, and wine coolers from your fridge, you'll have lots of extra room for a cut watermelon (my favorite fruit), cherries, apples, carrots, cucumbers, and hummus.

Even if your habits have been in motion for years, it isn't too late to change them, and it all starts with you, oh, Brave Parent. Making healthy decisions for you and your kiddos will reap rewards beyond your wildest imaginings.

CHAPTER 2 REFERENCES

Ali, F., Rehman, H., Babayan, Z., Stapleton, D., & Joshi, D.-D. (2015). Energy drinks and their adverse health effects: A systematic review of the current evidence. *Postgraduate Medicine, 127*(3), 308–322. https://doi.org/10.1080/00325481.2015.1001712.

Benbow, D. H. (2020, October 7). *The fascinating tale of Gatorade's Indy beginnings: '99.9% of Indiana does not know this'.* The Indianapolis Star. Retrieved September 25, 2021, from https://www.indystar.com/story/sports/2020/10/06/fascinating-tale-gatorades-indy-beginnings/5873513002/.

CDC. (2021, March 11). *Get the facts: Sugar-sweetened beverages and consumption.* Centers for Disease Control and Prevention. Retrieved September 25, 2021, from https://www.cdc.gov/nutrition/data-statistics/sugar-sweetened-beverages-intake.html.

Center for Food Safety and Applied Nutrition. (2019). *Generally recognized as safe (GRAS).* U.S. Food and Drug Administration. Retrieved September 26, 2021, from https://www.fda.gov/food/food-ingredients-packaging/generally-recognized-safe-gras.

Curtis, V. (2018, December 6). *Sugar in sports drinks.* University of Iowa Stead Family Children's Hospital. Retrieved September 25, 2021, from https://uichildrens.org/health-library/sugar-sports-drinks#:~:text=A%2032%2Dounce%20sports%20drink,amount%20-for%20kids%20and%20teenagers.

Das, A., & Chakraborty, R. (2016). Sweeteners: Classification, sensory and health effects. *Encyclopedia of Food and Health*, 234–240. https://doi.org/10.1016/b978-0-12-384947-2.00677-2

Drewnowski, A., & Bellisle, F. (2007). Liquid calories, sugar, and body weight. *The American Journal of Clinical Nutrition, 85*(3), 651–661. https://doi.org/10.1093/ajcn/85.3.651.

Dwyer, M. (2011, February 15). *Moderate alcohol intake may decrease men's risk for type 2 diabetes.* News. Retrieved September 26, 2021, from https://www.hsph.harvard.edu/news/features/moderate-alcohol-intake-may-decrease-mens-risk-for-type-2-diabetes/.

Fryar, C. D., Carroll, M. D., & Ogden, C. L. (2018, September 5). *Products - health e stats - prevalence of overweight and obesity among children and adolescents aged 2–19 years: United States, 1963–1965 through 2013–2014.* Centers for Disease Control and Prevention. Retrieved September 26, 2021, from https://www.cdc.gov/nchs/data/hestat/obesity_child_15_16/obesity_child_15_16.htm.

Honkala, S., Honkala, E., Tynjälä, J., & Kannas, L. (1999). Use of xylitol chewing gum among Finnish schoolchildren. *Acta Odontologica Scandinavica, 57*(6), 306–309. https://doi.org/10.1080/000163599428526.

Hutchinson, A. (2011). *Which comes First, cardio or weights?: Fitness myths, training truths, and other surprising discoveries from the science of Exercise.* HarperCollins.

Islam, S., & Indrajit, M. (2012). Effects of xylitol on blood glucose, glucose tolerance, serum insulin and lipid profile in a type 2 diabetes model of Rats. *Annals of Nutrition and Metabolism, 61*(1), 57–64. https://doi.org/10.1159/000338440.

Jorge, K. (2003). Soft drinks | chemical composition. *Encyclopedia of Food Sciences and Nutrition,* 5346–5352. https://doi.org/10.1016/b0-12-227055-x/01101-9.

Lustig, R. H. (2021). *Metabolical: The lure and the lies of processed food, nutrition, and Modern Medicine.* HarperWave, an imprint of HarperCollinsPublishers.

Pepino, M. Y. (2015). Metabolic effects of non-nutritive sweeteners. *Physiology & Behavior, 152,* 450–455. https://doi.org/10.1016/j.physbeh.2015.06.024.

Salli, K., Lehtinen, M. J., Tiihonen, K., & Ouwehand, A. C. (2019). Xylitol's Health Benefits Beyond Dental Health: A comprehensive review. *Nutrients, 11*(8), 1813. https://doi.org/10.3390/nu11081813.

SAMHSA, C. for B. H. S. and Q. (2013). *Update on emergency department visits involving Energy Drinks: A continuing public health concern.* The DAWN Report: Update on Emergency Department Visits Involving Energy Drinks: A Continuing Public Health Concern. Retrieved September 26, 2021, from https://www.samhsa.gov/data/

sites/default/files/DAWN126/DAWN126/sr126-energy-drinks-use.htm.

Shankar, P., Ahuja, S., & Sriram, K. (2013). Non-nutritive sweeteners: Review and update. *Nutrition, 29*(11-12), 1293–1299. https://doi.org/10.1016/j.nut.2013.03.024.

Sharp, G. (2010, October 25). *Changing soda serving sizes - sociological images.* Sociological Images Changing Soda Serving Sizes Comments. Retrieved September 25, 2021, from https://thesocietypages.org/socimages/2010/10/25/changing-soda-serving-sizes/.

Tabbers, M. M., DiLorenzo, C., Berger, M. Y., Faure, C., Langendam, M. W., Nurko, S., Staiano, A., Vandenplas, Y., & Benninga, M. A. (2014, February). *Evaluation and treatment of functional constipation in infants and children: Evidence-based recommendations from Espghan and Naspghan.* Journal of pediatric gastroenterology and nutrition. Retrieved September 25, 2021, from https://pubmed.ncbi.nlm.nih.gov/24345831/.

Trotter, J. K. (2013, October 30). *Americans drink 44 gallons of soda per year.* The Atlantic. Retrieved September 25, 2021, from https://www.theatlantic.com/national/archive/2013/03/americans-drink-44-gallons-soda-year/317523/.

Vandenberg, L. N., Maffini, M. V., Sonnenschein, C., Rubin, B. S., & Soto, A. M. (2009). Bisphenol-A and the Great Divide: A review of controversies in the field of endocrine disruption. *Endocrine Reviews, 30*(1), 75–95. https://doi.org/10.1210/er.2008-0021.

WHO. (2015, March 4). *Guideline: Sugars intake for adults and children.* World Health Organization. Retrieved September 25, 2021, from https://www.who.int/publications/i/item/9789241549028.

WHO. (2021, June 9). *Fact sheets - malnutrition.* World Health Organization. Retrieved September 25, 2021, from https://www.who.int/news-room/fact-sheets/detail/malnutrition.

Yew, D. (2020, October 25). *What is the prevalence of caffeine toxicity in the US?* Latest Medical News, Clinical Trials, Guidelines - Today on Medscape. Retrieved September 21, 2021, from https://

www.medscape.com/answers/821863-124341/what-is-the-prevalence-of-caffeine-toxicity-in-the-us.

Zeratsky, K. (2020, March 4). *Fruit juice: Good or bad for kids?* Mayo Clinic. Retrieved September 25, 2021, from https://www.mayoclinic.org/healthy-lifestyle/childrens-health/expert-answers/fruit-juice/faq-20058024.

CHAPTER THREE

digest

SUPPORT THE BUGS IN YOUR KID'S GUT ... OR THEIR GUT WILL BUG THEM

INTRODUCTION

W e've spent some time talking about food and drinks, so let's talk about how we digest them and why this is important. A number of gastrointestinal (GI) dysfunctions have increased in prevalence and become a huge focus in science and medicine these days. Acid reflux, inflammatory bowel disease, irritable bowel syndrome, ulcerative colitis, leaky gut, and other digestive disorders remain the hotspots in gut microbiome research.

What's to blame for the surge in prevalence? The science suggests that processed foods (especially fatty foods, fast foods, junk foods, fried foods, and hot/spicy foods) are blameworthy. But there are other identified culprits such as overuse of antibiotics, increasing prevalence of C-section delivery, over-sanitizing of our living environments, and stress. Even if your child doesn't ordinarily have GI challenges, please read on to learn how to make Brave Parent decisions so they don't have GI challenges in the future. What we know is that maintaining a healthy gut has become a continual challenge in today's world.

As a total health *dentist,* I frequently ask my patients about digestive issues, especially when I see chronic inflammation or fungal overgrowth in the mouth. It's astounding how many people suffer silently from chronic GI distress such as reflux, burping, bloating, nausea, diarrhea, constipation, gut pain, or bloody stools. They usually bear those burdens privately, but as with any chronic inflammatory conditions, these symptoms can be horrific to live with! What's really going on here? And why are these trends not slated to change anytime soon? Perhaps more importantly, how can we recognize warning signs in children before they escalate to bigger issues? In exploring these answers, let's start with the basics.

3.1 THE PURPOSE OF THE TUBE

Think of your digestive tract as a super long inner tube, with a surface area of about 2,700 square feet—about the size of a tennis court. It extends from the opening of your lips, where your food and drinks enter your piehole, to your pooper, where the unused waste comes out. The walls of the tube also serve as a permeable barrier, trying to keep your gut bacteria from invading the rest of the body. (When that fails, we have that upward-trending condition called *leaky gut.*) We are being bombarded with evidence that what happens, or doesn't happen, within that conduit is a major determinant to our overall health.

For the benefit of all our cells, the foods we consume (*macro*nutrients) have to be unpacked into usable particles (*micro*nutrients). It is the gut's job to do the unpacking, properly absorb the good stuff, and effectively discard the bad. To do that well, we must each have a massive population of microbes (bacteria, viruses, and fungi) residing within the tube. Our all-inclusive bug population is called the *microbiota,* or, as often used interchangeably, the *microbiome.*

"

There is a mountain of evidence that **microbial diversity** within the microbiome is the

key to health.

In other words, the more families of **helpful bugs** we host, the

better our digestion,

and the more protection we have from harmful bugs.

"

There is a mountain of evidence that microbial *diversity* within the microbiome is the key to health. In other words, the more families of helpful bugs we host, the better our digestion, and the more protection we have from harmful bugs.

Unfortunately, our Western, processed-food diet is associated with low microbial diversity. The microbiome of children who eat diets that are high in sugar, animal fat, and refined grains have markedly lower diversity than children who eat whole foods. Increasing the variety of plants kids consume is emerging as the most critical factor in restoring microbial diversity.

We sometimes forget that the mouth is the upper part of the digestive tract. Chewing food and mixing it with saliva, containing all its electrolytes and enzymes, begins the digestive process. The microbiome of the mouth differs from the gut, the vagina, and the skin. All four have a unique display of bacterial species. In the mouth alone, we've currently identified between 750 and 1,500 strains, depending on the diet, age, and geographic location. Incidentally, current genome sequencing research suggests there are thousands more still unidentified.

3.2 ALLERGIES AND AUTOIMMUNE DEFICIENCIES

Bacteria, viruses, and fungi ... oh my! Bugs always seem to freak us out—whether they're mosquitoes, spiders, and bees in the backyard or the microscopic variety living on us and in us. COVID-19 certainly heightened our bug anxiety. I've never seen so much hand sanitizer and surface disinfectant in my life! It's the true definition of overkill! Stay tuned, Brave Parents. There's more to come on the whens, whys, and how-tos of handwashing.

It's mind-blowing to think that for every human cell, we carry more than TEN microscopic bugs along for the ride. The ratio is 1:1 for bacteria and 10:1 favoring viruses. That varies between individuals, but the more assorted your bug population, the healthier you are presumed to be. And vice versa! This should come as no surprise because it is just as we observe in nature. Forests, lakes, oceans, and other wildlife habitats flourish with a wide diversity of life-forms. When you see the lack of diversity, you witness firsthand a suffering habitat.

When it comes to a deficient microbiome, there is a new epidemic in today's world. We've experienced an explosion of chronic, noncommunicable diseases (NCDs), thought to be primarily from the *significant decrease* in gut microbe populations over the past fifty years. There's a heap of good research pinning the big rise in allergies, asthma, autoimmune deficiencies, inflammatory bowel diseases, autism, diabetes, certain types of cancer, and even obesity on this deficit.

Genetics isn't believed to play as significant a role because our genetic makeup certainly hasn't changed much in fifty years, so it doesn't explain how food allergies have skyrocketed. According to the CDC, we've experienced a 50% increase between 1997 and 2011. Now one in every twenty kids has a food allergy. A child with an allergic reaction visits the emergency department every three minutes in the US. The most common food allergens for children are wheat, eggs, milk, peanuts, tree nuts, fish, shellfish, strawberries, sesame, and soy.

It's hard for doctors to keep up with the changing recommendations for allergy prevention and treatment. They are often challenged to give advice on how to introduce these foods. In 2000, the American Academy of Pediatrics (AAP) agreed that we should delay the introduction of cow's milk until age one, eggs until age two, and shellfish, fish, peanuts, and tree nuts until age three.

But in 2008 the pendulum began to swing the other way. It was determined that the current guidelines were ineffective, and maybe even contributing to the worsening pediatric allergy crisis. A recent landmark study showed children who received a delayed introduction to peanuts had a higher chance of developing an allergy compared to children who received an intro to peanuts between four and seven months.

Hence, the new recommendations by the American Academy of Allergy, Asthma & Immunology (AAAAI), Canadian Paediatric Society (CPS), and Canadian Society of Allergy and Clinical Immunology (CSACI) all agree that allergenic foods should be introduced like other whole foods. Present them one at a time, gradually, in small quantities, starting at four to six months (soon after vegetables and meats), and ideally before they are seven months old.

Today it's a better-known concept that the increase in food allergies also has to do with a lack of exposure to early-life microbes.

In the coming chapters, we will dig deeper into the root causes (and solutions) of our microbial inadequacy: antibiotic use, processed foods, C-sections, decreased connection to the outdoors, over-sanitization of our environment (i.e., commercial dishwashers, hot clothing driers, over-sanitization of surfaces), and a lack of agricultural diversity. Sadly, 75% of our food comes from only twelve plant species and five animal species.

3.3 PRE-BIRTH GUT AND C-SECTIONS

Before birth, your baby has a relatively sterile gut. The newest research suggests they have some bacteria populating their digestive tract even while they are in the womb but nothing like the rich population of bacteria they collect if they're lucky enough to be born through their mom's vaginal tract. Entering the world facedown, mouth-open, they get a whopping inoculation of mom's vaginal secretions and feces in their mouths and on their skin.

Next, as they nuzzle up to suckle mom's breast, they're exposed to mom's skin. All three of mom's microbiomes enrich a child's early gut. These new microscopic friends ready your baby to digest breast milk that will be produced within a few days. This all seems so miraculous to me!

> It's *mind-blowing* to think that for every human cell, **we carry more than TEN microscopic bugs** along for the ride. The ratio is 1:1 for bacteria and 10:1 favoring viruses. That varies between individuals, but the more assorted your bug population, the healthier you are presumed to be. And *vice versa*!

A baby who enters the world through a C-section, is considered less fortunate for bypassing his mom's rich gut bacteria. As a result, the mouth and gut become populated more haphazardly over time. Many C-section babies are slower to acquire the microbiome diversity indicative of health. As a result, they are associated with a higher incidence of digestive dysfunction that can last well into adulthood. Other studies have linked cesarean babies with an increased risk of childhood asthma and eczema.

The US CDC reports that approximately 32% of the 10,000 US babies born every day are by cesarean delivery. That's well above what the WHO considers the ideal between 10% and 15%.

Even though C-section poses higher risk of blood clots, infections, and long recovery times for mom, these numbers seem to have experienced steady increase over the past couple decades. The Natality data file from National Vital Statistics System shows that the cesarean rate rose by a whopping 53% from 1996 to 2007 for all mothers in all age and racial categories.

My patient Maurica Cox, an experienced OB nurse, speaks to this:

"A big reason for our increased C-section rates has to do with the declining health of our society. Our rates of obesity, heart disease, and additional comorbidities have significantly increased the risk of complications during pregnancy and delivery. All of these factors have played tribute to our increased C-section rate. If we became healthier as a population, it would have a positive impact on not just mode of delivery but also our infant mortality rate."

There is also a list of speculative reasons for the rise in C-sections including a desire for scheduling convenience, financial gain for the doc and medical facility, a culture of impatience, and the risk of litigation from possible negative outcomes of a difficult delivery. In your personal effort to avoid C-section, unless truly medically necessary, you'll want to have that discussion with your doctor ahead of time.

" Before birth, your baby has a relatively **sterile gut**. The newest research suggests they have some bacteria populating their digestive tract even while they are in the *womb* but nothing like the **rich population of bacteria** they collect if they're lucky enough to be born through their mom's vaginal tract.

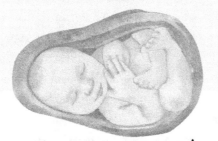

Entering the world facedown, mouth-open, they get a whopping **inoculation** of mom's vaginal secretions and feces in their mouths and on their skin. **"**

3.4 INFANT MICROBIOTA DEVELOPMENT

When human babies are born their gut is immature and can handle only breast milk. Mom's milk has the perfect combination of 10% proteins, 30% fat, and 60% carbohydrates. Along with micronutrients (and even some of the mom's microbiota) this is the perfect recipe for the first four to six months while the baby's intestines are maturing enough to process some solid food. Meanwhile, your baby is developing trillions of microbial cells to colonize the entire surface of her gut lining. It is the same with your mouth. (See section 7.4 on Caries Disease in chapter 7 Chew and Smile.)

Breast milk is also the best source of nutrition for a baby's developing microbiota. Numerous studies document better health outcomes for breast milk-fed children, including reduced rates of infections, asthma, and obesity. And while the breast milk is like a magic potion, the *act* of breastfeeding is magic too. Sucking directly from a breast (versus a bottle) builds strong tongue and facial muscles which is critically beneficial in oral cavity and facial development. There's much more to come about the majesty of the suck in chapter 4 Breathe.

Breastfeeding correctly can be very natural, with your baby leading the way, but it can also be really difficult. For many moms, it's not as intuitive as it looks. Be patient the first few weeks, and by all means, consult an International Board Certified Lactation Consultant (IBCLC). Make sure your consultant evaluates your baby's tongue and lips for tethered tissues. Breastfeeding restrictions can be caused by an anterior or posterior tongue-tie or an upper lip-tie that might need to be released. If you are intent on breastfeeding, try to avoid giving bottles in the first few weeks to avoid nipple confusion. Consider cup feeding if you need to. (Learn more on lip- and tongue-ties and cup feeding in chapter 4 Breathe.)

Because mom's milk helps diversify the microbiota, the recommendation is for babies to enjoy at least four months of breastmilk, but if it's possible, keep it going as you introduce whole foods. There is sound evidence that baby's gut bacteria benefit from breastfeeding up to two years.

If you decide to feed your baby formula instead of breastmilk, you might want to bolster *good* gut bacteria that the baby is missing. Complementing baby formula with pediatric probiotics is proving to be a good idea, but the supplement needs to be of high quality and adequate diversity. To find the best quality probiotics, or probiotic-fortified formula, consult your pediatrician or nutritionist. I'll cover more on probiotics ahead in the section on antibiotics.

3.5 BABY'S FIRST FOODS

At about four to six months, you will start to introduce solid foods. Look for signs of readiness, including interest and their ability to swallow while sitting up. It helps to have a highchair that allows your baby to sit up straight. That posture also gives them better control over their arms and hands if you should try baby-led weaning (see the next section).

With the introduction of solid foods, we see a big change in the baby's microbiota. New strains of bacteria are continually introduced. Plant fiber (also called *prebiotics*) feed the bugs, and within a few months your little sweetheart's gut bacteria starts to acquire more diversity and resemble the microbiota of an adult. (Incidentally, prebiotics, despite the similarity in name to *probiotics*, is not bacteria, but food for beneficial bacteria to flourish.) Studies show that a one-year-old's gut is supporting about 60% more bacterial species than just seven months earlier!

In an adult we have somewhere between 300 and 1,000 identified bacterial strains with 99% coming from thirty to forty species. Remember, the more diverse the better.

Even if your baby is lucky enough to enter the world through a vaginal delivery, the newborn intestine is immature and not ready for real food. Notice that as the array of bacteria expands, your diaper changes become more "interesting."

Eating a wide variety of foods will increase diversity, and it's especially important in the first two to three years. You can begin to introduce solid foods at about four to six months, when they can sit up without support. Introduce one food at a time and in small tastes. You're aiming for a wholesome, varied diet, rich in fiber and low in animal fat and sugar.

Kids around the world start with *very* different first foods, but in our culture, we have tended toward a processed, single-grain cereal such as rice. For microbiome diversity, present a variety of refined whole grains such as whole wheat, oats, rye, barley, millet, maize, and brown rice.

Remember that, as a population, fiber is our number one deficiency, and leaning heavily on a single processed grain, like rice cereal, will fail to boost the developing microbiota.

Also introduce legumes such as lentils, beans, and peas, which are high in fiber and can be easily mashed with a fork. Include vegetables in all meals including nontraditional root vegetables such as sweet potatoes and parsnips. Another way to boost microbial diversity is to introduce naturally fermented foods like kefir and yogurt (but avoid sweetened processed yogurt, as it can hide as much added sugar as a can of cola).

At age six months, iron levels may start to decrease. To prevent iron deficiency anemia (associated with brain development problems), you'll want to introduce meat or meat alternatives such as eggs, tofu, legumes, or iron-fortified cereal.

Again, you can follow the AAAAI recommendations (above) on introducing allergenic foods, but stay up to date on the newest research and recommendations in this arena as it is ever evolving.

The bottom line: throughout your child's life, nothing will influence their healthy microbiota more than the foods they eat. Make diversity and variety within all four food groups the central theme of your kitchen strategy.

66

The bottom line: throughout your child's life, nothing will influence their **healthy microbiota** more than the *foods they eat.*

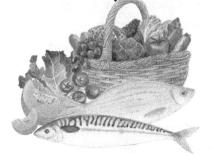

Make **diversity and variety** within **all four food groups** the central theme of your kitchen *strategy*.

99

3.6 BABY-LED WEANING (BLW)

Beginning in the UK and New Zealand around 2005, this approach to feeding babies has continued to grow in popularity in the US.

It's an alternative method of adding *complementary* whole foods to your baby's diet of breast milk or formula. Instead of spoon-feeding a puree of food, you can introduce easy-to-grasp finger foods that are soft enough to be easily squished between your fingers. Your baby's independent exploration will include seeing, smelling, licking, sucking, and feeling the texture of the food before continuing on to eat it.

BLW helps the development of age-appropriate oral motor control while enhancing the eating experience to be more positive and interactive. It also supports the development of self-feeding because your baby gets to be in charge of what goes in their mouth, of what consistency, and when.

It still amazes me that a healthy newborn has the complex ability to suck, swallow, and breathe, simultaneously getting their nutrition while protecting their airway. That pattern is innate and thus considered a reflex. But the oral motor patterns necessary for eating solid foods are learned, not reflexive. These include tongue lateralization, tongue elevation, and chewing.

Swallowing pureed foods is much like swallowing another liquid. Baby-led weaning, however, helps develop the oral motor patterns required for mature chewing and swallowing.

One of the many reasons this trend is growing in popularity is that it's easy. If you are already eating a balanced diet of whole foods, you can easily modify your foods to share with your baby. So, when is a baby ready to start BLW? The American Academy of Pediatrics (AAP) suggests it's when:

- They've doubled their birth weight (at least).
- They can hold their head up well and are starting to sit up

unsupported.
- They show signs of interest in food (watching you eat, reaching for food when you're eating, etc.).
- When you feed them, they can move the food around in their mouths, rather than spit it right out.

To learn more, take a look at the book *Baby-Led Weaning: The Essential Guide* by Dr. Gill Rapley and Tracey Murkett.

3.7 ANTIBIOTICS: THE ANGEL AND THE DEVIL

In the pre-antibiotic age, prior to 1945, a simple infection could be life-threatening. In fact, during the American Civil War, more people died from infection than bullets. For children and adults, many common bacterial infections escalated rapidly to death. Then along came the most miraculous classification of drugs ever invented. Antibiotics transformed the way we treated infectious diseases. Manufacturing and distribution were ratcheted up during World War II, and it didn't stop there.

By the time I was in dental school, they were almost as common as candy. I was told by one of my dental school instructors (circa 1983) about antibiotics, "Never worry about prescribing too many or too much (antibiotics). No one has ever overdosed on the stuff."

My how times have changed! We absolutely *do* need to worry about the overuse of antibiotics, on a personal level and a global health level.

The problem is basically twofold.

First, antibiotics are losing their punch as the antibiotic-resistant genes in the bacteria themselves are becoming more widespread. Have you heard the term *superbugs*? These are robust antibiotic-resistant strains like MRSA, VRE, and MDR TB. Clearly in response to our massive use of antibiotics, resistance is now arising within a year or two, often making the newly introduced antibiotics obsolete within three to five years. As a response, most pharmaceutical companies have chipped away at the budget allocated for their antibiotic discovery divisions. With fewer new drugs emerging and the ones we have no longer working, we will soon face the fears your great-grandparents did.

In fact, the WHO considers antimicrobial resistance a serious threat that is no longer just a prediction. It is happening right now and has the potential to affect anyone of any age and in any country.

The second problem is that antibiotics don't just kill the nasty bacteria we're targeting. They kill a massive supply of protective bacteria in our gut along the way. That's why you notice your kiddos' poops suddenly change consistency when they start an antibiotic. Unfortunately, it doesn't bounce right back after the course is completed. It might take months. In the worst-case scenario, we can develop a potentially deadly infection called *C. Diff*. More commonly, we can cause permanent extinction of many entire families of bugs. In fact, our gut bug diversity is about half of what our ancestors had, and this depletion is wreaking havoc with our immune systems. If you're interested in more on this subject, read Dr. Martin Blaser's *Missing Microbes: How the Overuse of Antibiotics is Fueling Our Modern Plagues*.

There are individual health risks, too, even beyond the slight possibility of a serious allergic reaction. It has been shown that multiple courses of antibiotics during your baby's first year significantly increases their risk of asthma. Then there's the increased risk of pediatric obesity and type 2 diabetes. Even short pulses of antibiotic use alter your kiddo's nutrient uptake and promotes weight gain.

Astute physicians, dentists, NPs, and PAs are aware of these destructions and are trying to be more "responsible" by not prescribing antibiotics right off the bat. For example, 75% of kids get an ear infection (otitis media) at some point, and the recommendation is to wait 48–72 hours, especially if your kiddo is older than six months, is otherwise healthy, and has mild symptoms. About two-thirds of mild earache cases resolve without antibiotics.

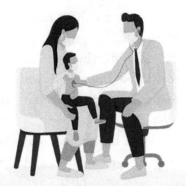

" Be your kids' *Brave Parent* and keep their future health in mind. That means choosing good docs that are **future-health focused** (not just disease reactive) and **trusting their judgment**. Don't push them to prescribe **antibiotics** against their better *judgment.* "

For a sore throat, your doc may ask you to wait for the results of a strep test before prescribing. There are many viral infections that can stimulate a sore throat, for example the common cold, in which case bacterial antibiotics are useless.

But many moms and dads literally plead for a prescription. I get it! If your child has a sore throat or earache, you want desperately to fend off pain and a more serious systemic infection, such as rheumatic fever, at the get-go.

It's important to choose a health care team you trust and give them the leadership role. As a dentist, I can tell you it's always a dilemma. I have a hard time convincing my local oral surgeons when extracting wisdom teeth *not* to prescribe a *preventive* antibiotic for a healthy child, unless warranted by existing infection. (As an important aside, I *definitely do not* want them to automatically prescribe a post-surgical opioid pain killer. Since it's often a teen's first taste of an opioid, it can stimulate a euphoric feeling they might be enticed to repeat.)

So, despite the widespread knowledge that antibiotics can, in the long run, be dangerous, US medical and dental professionals still write two antibiotic prescriptions per person, per year! We, as health care professionals, need your help in this undertaking.

Be your kids' Brave Parent and keep their future health in mind. That means choosing good docs that are future-health focused (not just disease reactive) and trusting their judgment. Don't push them to prescribe antibiotics against their better judgment.

When your doctor does prescribe, you can help prevent microbial ruin by providing a pediatric probiotic supplement a couple times a day. If you give your child the probiotic simultaneously, the antibiotic will wipe out the good microbes, too, so it's suggested you give them (usually in liquid form) one to two hours *after* the medicine. Pediatric probiotics should include at least *Saccharomyces boulardii* (a yeast probiotic) and *Lactobacillus rhamnosus GG* in order to affront diarrhea and a risk of *C. diff* colitis (infection of the colon).

I would be remiss if I didn't add that 80% of antibiotics sold in the US today (that is, 80% of the nineteen million pounds per year) are sold to feed livestock and transferred to people who consume the treated meat and dairy products.

Antibiotics for livestock were introduced to fend off communicable infection among the herd, but the result was interesting. It became apparent that feeding animals low levels of antibiotics caused them to fatten up quickly. That fattened the profit margins, too, and as such, it became common practice.

Pediatric obesity and premature breast development in girls *and* boys have now been linked with a steady consumption of antibiotics in milk and meat. For all these reasons, try your best to buy antibiotic-free, grass-fed animals, and proportion the meat and dairy as garnishes to the meal, with the veggies as the mainstay.

3.8 ANTIBIOTICS FOR DENTAL INFECTIONS

A toothache deserves your immediate attention. Dental caries (cavities) is the most prevalent disease among children worldwide (See chapter 7 Chew and Smile). The trauma from decay (or a filling to treat the decay) can lead all the way to pulp death, excruciating pain, abscess, and facial swelling. In that case, it usually results in your child's dentist removing the tooth right away in order to avoid the need for antibiotics. Unless there is significant facial swelling, a localized infection will resolve soon after the sick tooth is removed.

Calling Brave Parents! It might be up to you to advocate for immediate removal rather than an antibiotic prescription to reduce the swelling before the extraction. I say that because the dental profession is lagging in its response to the antibiotic crisis. A large 2018 look-back study revealed that from 1996 to 2013, physician prescribing declined 18.2%. Now that's progress! Unfortunately, dental prescribing increased 62.2% during that same time, and dentistry's proportionate contribution increased from 6.7% to 11.3% of all antibiotic prescriptions.

"

Pediatric **obesity**
and **premature breast
development** in girls and boys
have now been linked with a
steady **consumption of
antibiotics** in milk and meat.

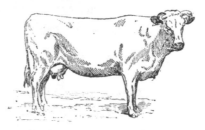

For all these reasons, try your
best to buy **antibiotic-free**,
grass-fed animals, and
proportion the *meat and dairy*
as garnishes to the meal, with
the **veggies as the mainstay**.

"

Most of the *unnecessary* prescriptions were thought to center around medicating for toothaches and dental abscesses to buy time while delaying or referring to specialists for extractions. Other plausible reasons listed were unwarranted preventive antibiotics for extraction of wisdom teeth, preventive antibiotics for placement of dental implants, and ignoring the updated guidelines calling for far less antibiotic premedication for patients with valvular heart disease and joint replacements.

For *all* health care professionals, antibiotic prescribing should be reviewed to make sure we stay compliant with current guidelines. If we do that, most of us will find opportunities to prescribe less often and for shorter durations.

3.9 VACCINATIONS

This is a difficult section to write because we have never seen greater pushback on vaccination than in the fight to gain herd immunity over COVID-19. I have never been a fan of bombarding your baby with more than a dozen vaccine shots for immunity to about twenty dangerous pathogens, all before the age of fifteen months. The intensity of that onboarding schedule remains controversial among my wellness-focused friends (i.e., the docs in my Wellness and Prevention Study Club).

That said, all it would take is your child's serious illness or death from the intentional omission of a single vaccination, and you might suffer a lifetime of regret. Vaccinations have muted so many once-deadly communicable diseases such as polio, measles, mumps, rubella, diphtheria, tetanus, pertussis, hepatitis B, hepatitis A, and influenzas. They are the very reason our society has evolved to such a low infant mortality rate. To appreciate this, let's turn back the hands of time through the story of my eighty-four-year-old patient, Walt, a retired scientist.

In the beginning of COVID, Walt came in for a dental visit, and I asked how he was doing with his newfound isolation and fear of infectivity. He casually shrugged and said:

"It's just a matter of time. We will slay this! You see, at the age of nine, I contracted polio, which is how I lost the use of my left leg. I was quarantined, away from my family, in an infectious disease unit in the hospital. There was an open bed next to me where they brought in another young man. At first, they didn't know what he was sick with, but when I got rubella, they found out!

"I eventually left the hospital with no use of my leg and a heart defect from rubella. Then, I got mumps at age eleven. First on the right side, then three months later on the left side. Mumps put me back in the hospital again, fighting for my life. But look around in today's world ... these are diseases kids don't even know about today, thanks to vaccines."

Then he reassured me again, "So don't worry kid. We'll get this vaccine, and I bet it will be sooner than you think."

I've repeated that prophetic story countless times because it put it all in perspective for me.

Even though the risks are minuscule, it's possible for an individual to have an unwanted side effect from a vaccine, and we fear that for our children even more than ourselves. I still get questions about vaccines being linked to the rise in autism spectrum disorder (ASD). It's just not founded. Highly qualitative and quantitative science has irrefutably debunked that postulation. If you want an entirely scientific and historical perspective on this, be sure to hear Dr. Peter Attia's podcast *The Drive,* where he interviews Dr. Brian Deer. It's called "A tale of scientific fraud—exposing Andrew Wakefield and the origin of the belief that vaccines cause autism."

So, what exactly is a vaccine and how does it work? It's either a weakened version of the *actual* virus or bacteria (called live-attenuated) or a laboratory-replicated fragment of the virus. When introduced to our body, we miraculously build natural protection to the replica—an army of soldiers, so to speak, armed and ready to fend off the *real* bug.

If you've ever felt a little icky for a couple days following a vaccination, it's because your body recognizes the resemblance of the bug, and you're busy building that army of defense. Maybe you even experienced that with your recent COVID-19 shot.

Not unlike some other viruses, COVID *vaccination immunity* offers longer and more effective results than *convalescent immunity* (the response you get after fighting the disease itself). That's because vaccination produces greater numbers of circulating antibodies than natural infection. As an added bonus, vaccination stimulates memory B cells faster than disease does, helping us fight even the viral variants we see cropping up.

Bugs that harm humans jump from person to person. They need a *host*. Without enough human bodies to infect, they virtually disappear from our population. That concept is called *herd immunity*.

With an outbreak like COVID-19, we need to reach an estimated 80% population immunity for that to happen. That means somewhere around 80% of us will need to have immunity—*at the same time*. Until we get there, this bug will do what it naturally does —*adapt* in order to survive beyond the vaccine. The Delta variant of the coronavirus is only the first example of an adaptation. It is more contagious than the first but luckily, most vaccinated people are either asymptomatic or have very mild symptoms if they contract the Delta variant.

Personally, I found it tragic that most of my patients' opinions about the COVID vaccine were not shaped by high-quality studies. In the US most of our opinions were predominately shaped by either politically slanted news channels or our most memorable social media messages. Meanwhile conspiracy theories continue to abound, and some of them include the COVID vaccines.

I have *real* news for you though. Clean, hard science doesn't care what you believe! Good data continues to emerge, and we have to be willing to change our minds in response to valid data, or we will live isolated, masked, and with intermittent shutdowns from outbreaks and variants.

I know it's frustrating that the dialogue changes as we learn more, but it's up to each of us to allow our *beliefs* to be influenced by the most recent, well-scrutinized studies, published in peer-reviewed scientific journals. Not small, shallow studies that benefit from financial gain or social or political glorification.

That's a tall order. The challenge is, how the heck does a nonscience person gain access to current studies in peer-reviewed journals? Through all of this, I grew acutely aware of our country's science illiteracy. And I noticed how ill-trusted even the most high-integrity studies/scholars have become, along with their inability to quell people's fears.

I remain concerned that our science-skeptical culture might dismiss the enormous body of knowledge about vaccinations in general, their historical magic, and how profoundly they've saved kids' lives.

3.10 IS IT BETTER TO BE CLEAN OR DIRTY?

Even before the COVID-19 pandemic, most US families lived in homes where every fork is washed (and sanitized) in a hot dishwasher, every T-shirt is washed and dried (and sanitized) in a hot washer/dryer, every drop of water is chlorinated (sanitized) or stored in plastic bottles, and even our bodies and hair are washed in hot soapy water multiple times a week. Since the pandemic, alcohol-based hand *sanitizer* and multipurpose home cleaner sales both skyrocketed. We have become fixated on sterilizing our environments, and many are touting it, saying, "It's about time we got serious about cleanliness."

When it comes to your child's microbial diversity and fortifying our immune systems, these accepted "health practices" are simply ... not so great. Our kids were already starving for connection to the outdoors as well as face-to-face play, and this pandemic took us 180 degrees in the opposite direction.

66

Calling all *Brave Parents:* Prevailing over our obsession to sanitize, it's important to *explain* to your children the idea that their bodies are a good home to hundreds of families of helpful, **healing bugs**. And to keep these little critters happy we need to feed them what they like—plenty of vegetables (fiber). **Food for bugs** is what we are now calling **prebiotics**.

99

If you look up *germophobia* in Wikipedia, it is described as an obsessive-compulsive disorder and typified by these signs and symptoms:

- Excessive handwashing
- An avoidance of locations that might contain a high presence of germs
- A fear of physical contact, especially with strangers
- Excessive effort dedicated to cleaning and sanitizing one's environment
- A refusal to share personal items
- A fear of becoming ill

Does that sound familiar? Welcome to life amidst a viral pandemic! COVID-19 is a scary bug that had us ALL on high alert. Now, post-vaccination, I'm curious about the lasting impact of our germophobic mindset as I'm witnessing many families not easing up on these now ingrained sanitization habits.

Calling all Brave Parents: Prevailing over our obsession to sanitize, it's important to explain to your children the idea that their bodies are a good home to hundreds of families of *helpful, healing* bugs. And to keep these little critters happy we need to feed them what they like—plenty of vegetables (fiber). Food for bugs is what we are now calling *pre*biotics.

At the end of the day, we truly are social beings—wired for human connection, for love, and for belonging. These needs are most often demonstrated through regular gestures of touch: handshakes, hugs, kisses, and hand-holding. Demonstrate this often, even if you grew up with parents who didn't.

And what is more, we are all yearning for reconnection to nature. Be the Brave Parent and steer your kids toward regular, unstructured outdoor playtime. Read on to learn how it will feed their souls and fuel their microbiome!

"

How soon can your
baby meet your **pup**?

The *younger* the better!

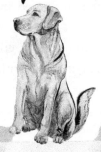

There is good **evidence** that
mom's exposure to a **dog** during
pregnancy and **baby's exposure**
during early life **decrease**
allergies and **eczema by 30%**
and asthma by 20%.

3.11 OUTDOOR PLAY AND INDOOR PETS

Kids are wired for playing outside, in and amongst nature, exploring fields, waterways, and forests. And for playing with insects, watching birds, and petting our dogs, cats, bunnies, and chickens. (So, by the way, are adults!)

If you were raised forty or more years ago, you might remember rushing home to finish your homework, *not* so you could have more time for computer gaming or social media surfing, but so you could *play outside* until you were summoned indoors for a bath, tooth-brushing, and bedtime.

Getting down-to-earth and dirty is critical for helping us with microbial diversity and fortifying our immune systems. Teach kids that it's okay to dig for worms, study caterpillars, pet farm animals, and dissect flowers, but they should avoid touching dead animals or animal feces (including their own).

Let your children explore the outdoors, and resist the urge to hand-sanitize until it's time to come in. Then offer soap and water, which is just as effective and does not force them to absorb alcohol or harsh chemicals through their skin. Antibacterial soaps are not beneficial over regular soap. And hand sanitizer should only be applied when there is not access to soap and water.

Beyond microbial diversity, being connected to nature is good for social and emotional restoration. For most people, natural environments are spiritually grounding. Intermingling with other living communities reminds your kiddos that they are each a small part of a larger environment. It offers a great opportunity to you to express some societal responsibility, emphasizing respect for and protection of our earth's natural habitats.

Living with pets in your household helps kids learn responsibility to and caring for another living being. But it can also help boost their immunity and reduce allergies. Multiple studies show this is true of dogs, but not cats. Dogs bring the outside environment in, which diversifies our microbiome, whereas cats tend to live indoors and poop in a litter box. Plus, a cat's feces, more often than a dog's, can carry parasites, so keep the litter box out of reach until your child is responsible enough to avoid playing in it.

Both dogs and cats offer companionship and sometimes protection, but when your dog snuggles up with your child and gives a lick on the face, appreciate the moment. It actually *helps* with microbial diversity and immunity.

How soon can your baby meet your pup? The younger the better! There is good evidence that mom's exposure to a dog during pregnancy and baby's exposure during early life decrease allergies and eczema by 30% and asthma by 20%.

I couldn't be happier for this news since my allergist (around 1970) advised just the opposite. To help with my fifty-two allergies and immune deficiencies, he insisted my parents get rid of my cats *and* my dog until I was older and stronger—and suggested even then I should never have a dog who sheds. I was absolutely heartbroken, and the hurt lasted for months. There is nothing like a child's bond to their beloved dog, especially a child who has chronic illness.

The future body of research on the human microbiota will be amazing. Stay tuned. The Human Microbiome Project is a large collection of research projects that together are proving to be a powerful driver of medical breakthroughs for decades to come. Soon, we are expected to use probiotic therapy for real-time cures to some of the most significant diseases and disorders we see today.

If you're still reading and this subject has captured your attention, you must read the important research-stacked book, *Let Them Eat Dirt: Saving Your Child from an Oversanitized World* by Arrieta and Finlay. (www.letthemeatdirt.com)

CONCLUSION

People with gut issues suffer in silence. But oh, how they suffer. One of my beloved nephews was dealt ulcerative colitis, an inflammatory bowel disease. During active episodes it's been painful, frightening, and a huge disruption in both his business career and personal life. My heart wanted to break when he described how anxious and distracted he was in business meetings because he would suddenly need to bolt to the nearest bathroom for an awful experience.

I can tell you first-hand that my nephew's nightmare has become more and more common. As I ask my new patients if they suffer from the litany of ugly symptoms, the stories that follow are often tales of fear, embarrassment, and trauma. I wish I could wave a magic wand to assure that none of these debilitating gut dysfunctions or diseases will make it onto your child's heath history, but once again, the magic lies mostly in your ability to ***prevent*** them.

Meanwhile, there is hope that targeted probiotic therapies will provide safe and effective remedies for some life-crippling GI disturbances. Let's all keep a keen eye on the developing body of research as the field of microbial gut health *explodes*! (Pardon the pun—I couldn't resist.)

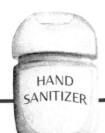

> Let your *children explore* the outdoors, and **resist the urge to hand-sanitize** until it's time to come in. Then offer **soap and water**, which is just as **effective** and does not force them to absorb alcohol or harsh chemicals through their skin. **Antibacterial soaps are not beneficial over regular soap**. And hand sanitizer should only be applied when there is not access to soap and water.

CHAPTER 3 REFERENCES

Abrams, E. M., & Becker, A. B. (2015, November 17). *Food introduction and allergy prevention in infants.* CMAJ : Canadian Medical Association journal = journal de l'Association medicale canadienne. Retrieved September 25, 2021, from https://www.ncbi.nlm.nih.gov/pmc/articles/PMC4646750/.

Ballard, O., & Morrow, A. L. (2013, February). *Human milk composition: Nutrients and bioactive factors.* Pediatric clinics of North America. Retrieved September 25, 2021, from https://www.ncbi.nlm.nih.gov/pmc/articles/PMC3586783/.

Begum, A. (2018). Antibiotics in dentistry-double-edged sword. *Open Access Journal of Dental Sciences, 3*(1). https://doi.org/10.23880/oajds-16000161.

Blaser, M. J. (2015). *Missing microbes: How the overuse of antibiotics is fueling our modern plagues.* Picador.

Brown, A., Jones, S. W., & Rowan, H. (2017). *Baby-led weaning: The evidence to date.* Current nutrition reports. Retrieved September 25, 2021, from https://www.ncbi.nlm.nih.gov/pmc/articles/PMC5438437/.

CDC. (2015, November 6). *Products - data briefs - number 121 - May 2013.* Centers for Disease Control and Prevention. Retrieved September 25, 2021, from https://www.cdc.gov/nchs/products/databriefs/db121.htm.

CDC. (2021, August 24). *When, what, and how to introduce Solid Foods.* Centers for Disease Control and Prevention. Retrieved September 25, 2021, from https://www.cdc.gov/nutrition/infantandtoddlernutrition/foods-and-drinks/when-to-introduce-solid-foods.html.

CDC. (2021, March 2). *FastStats - Births - method of delivery.* Centers for Disease Control and Prevention. Retrieved September 25, 2021, from https://www.cdc.gov/nchs/fastats/delivery.htm.

Chin, B., Chan, E. S., & Goldman, R. D. (2014, April). *Early expo-*

sure to food and food allergy in Children. Canadian family physician Medecin de famille canadien. Retrieved September 25, 2021, from https://www.ncbi.nlm.nih.gov/pmc/articles/PMC4046529/.

Cox, L. M., & Blaser, M. J. (2015, March). *Antibiotics in early life and obesity.* Nature reviews. Endocrinology. Retrieved September 25, 2021, from https://www.ncbi.nlm.nih.gov/pmc/articles/PMC4487629/.

Cruchet, S., Furnes, R., Maruy, A., Hebel, E., Palacios, J., Medina, F., Ramirez, N., Orsi, M., Rondon, L., Sdepanian, V., Xóchihua, L., Ybarra, M., & Zablah, R. A. (2015, June). *The use of probiotics in pediatric gastroenterology: A review of the literature and recommendations by Latin-American experts.* Paediatric drugs. Retrieved September 25, 2021, from https://www.ncbi.nlm.nih.gov/pmc/articles/PMC4454830/.

Deo, P. N., & Deshmukh, R. (2019). *Oral microbiome: Unveiling the fundamentals.* Journal of oral and maxillofacial pathology : JOMFP. Retrieved September 25, 2021, from https://www.ncbi.nlm.nih.gov/pmc/articles/PMC6503789/.

Finlay, B. B., & Arrieta, M.-C. (2017). *Let them eat dirt: Saving your child from an oversanitized world.* Windmill Books.

Fleischer, D. M., Chan, E. S., Venter, C., Spergel, J. M., Abrams, E. M., Stukus, D., Groetch, M., Shaker, M., & Greenhawt, M. (2020, November 26). *A consensus approach to the primary prevention of food allergy through nutrition: Guidance from the American Academy of Allergy, asthma, and Immunology; American College of Allergy, asthma, and immunology; and the Canadian Society for Allergy and Clinical Immunology.* The Journal of Allergy and Clinical Immunology: In Practice. Retrieved September 25, 2021, from https://www.sciencedirect.com/science/article/abs/pii/S2213219820312113?via%3Dihub.

Gould, D. (2019, September 30). *Introducing biodiversity: The intersection of Taste & Sustainability.* Food+Tech Connect. Retrieved September 25, 2021, from https://foodtechconnect.com/2019/01/07/biodiverse-food-intersection-taste-sustainability/#:~:text=About%2075%20per-cent%20of%20the,only%20eat%20150%20of%20them.

Helander, H. F., & Fändriks, L. (2014). *Surface area of the digestive tract - revisited.* Scandinavian journal of gastroenterology. Retrieved September 24, 2021, from https://pubmed.ncbi.nlm.nih.gov/24694282/.

Johnson, C. C., & Ownby, D. R. (2016). *Allergies and asthma: Do atopic disorders result from inadequate immune homeostasis arising from infant gut dysbiosis?* Expert review of clinical immunology. Retrieved September 25, 2021, from https://www.ncbi.nlm.nih.gov/pmc/articles/PMC4829075/.

Khan, I., Ullah, N., Zha, L., Bai, Y., Khan, A., Zhao, T., Che, T., & Zhang, C. (2019, August 13). *Alteration of gut microbiota in inflammatory bowel disease (IBD): Cause or consequence? IBD treatment targeting the gut microbiome.* Pathogens (Basel, Switzerland). Retrieved September 24, 2021, from https://www.ncbi.nlm.nih.gov/pmc/articles/PMC6789542/.

Lodge, C. J., Allen, K. J., Lowe, A. J., Hill, D. J., Hosking, C. S., Abramson, M. J., & Dharmage, S. C. (2012). *Perinatal cat and dog exposure and the risk of asthma and allergy in the urban environment: A systematic review of longitudinal studies.* Clinical & developmental immunology. Retrieved September 25, 2021, from https://www.ncbi.nlm.nih.gov/pmc/articles/PMC3251799/.

Loo, E. X. L., Sim, J. Z. T., Loy, S. L., Goh, A., Chan, Y. H., Tan, K. H., Yap, F., Gluckman, P. D., Godfrey, K. M., Van Bever, H., Lee, B. W., Chong, Y. S., Shek, L. P.-C., Koh, M. J. A., & Ang, S. B. (2017, May). *Associations between caesarean delivery and allergic outcomes: Results from the Gusto Study.* Annals of allergy, asthma & immunology : official publication of the American College of Allergy, Asthma, & Immunology. Retrieved September 25, 2021, from https://www.ncbi.nlm.nih.gov/pmc/articles/PMC5505471/.

Lynch, S. V., & Author Affiliations From the Division of Gastroenterology. (2016, December 15). *The human intestinal microbiome in health and disease: Nejm.* New England Journal of Medicine. Retrieved

September 25, 2021, from https://www.nejm.org/doi/full/10. 1056/NEJMra1600266.

Menacker, F., & Hamilton, B. E. (2010). *Recent trends in cesarean delivery in the United States.* NCHS data brief. Retrieved September 25, 2021, from https://pubmed.ncbi.nlm.nih.gov/20334736/.

Tobey, R. E. (2018, May 28). *Advances in medicine during wars: A Primer.* Foreign Policy Research Institute. Retrieved September 25, 2021, from https://www.fpri.org/article/2018/02/advances-medicine-wars-primer/.

CHAPTER FOUR
breathe

GROWING THE TONGUE BOX: IT'S THE SHAPE OF THINGS TO COME

INTRODUCTION

A human being can live for three weeks without food.

Three days without water.

But only three minutes without oxygen.

Oxygen! It's hands down our number one nutrient. Air quality is critical, and so is our body's healthy respiratory system. It allows us to sift through our ambient air, snatching up oxygen molecules to fuel every cell in our bodies.

I grew up an oxygen-starved kid, and that deeply etched memory has always haunted me. At twelve, when I began to learn how it felt to breathe like a normal person, I was determined never to go back there. Then a few years ago, I watched my mom struggle for breath as she lay suffocating from acute lymphoma that settled in her lungs. It seemed unbearable to witness.

I queried her pulmonologist, a friend of mine, for advice on how I might endure the experience of watching this person I deeply love slowly asphyxiate. I'll never forget his answer: "I wish I knew, Susan. Even after all the years I've treated patients, the thought of dying from a long, slow progression of oxygen deprivation just petrifies me."

Oxygen deprivation isn't normally so in-your-face like it was for me. But make no mistake, if you hang around a bunch of kids, you'll see it in subtle little sneaky manifestations, and it's critical to be aware of the signs so you can act when needed. I'll teach you how to look more closely at your tired, wired, ADHD, defiant, irritable, and chronically sick kids, to help Brave Parents overturn the root cause of their kids' behavior issues.

Many of these behavior issues are from sleep deprivation—the usual sidekick to pediatric airway dysfunction. Because SLEEP, both the quality and quantity of it, is so profoundly important to your child's health, it deserves a separate chapter (to follow). For now, just recognize that both *good breathing* and *good sleep* are essential for optimal health, and the lack of either (or both) are much more common in children than we ever realized.

The historic literature reports that only 5% of children have obstructive sleep apnea (OSA), but today's experts in airway and sleep medicine know *that* number doesn't tell the whole story.

Sleep-disordered breathing (SDB) in children is estimated to be 30–35% if you also count mouth breathing, flow limitations such as snoring, upper airway resistance syndrome (UARS), obstructive sleep apnea (OSA), chronic congestion from allergies, chronic upper respiratory infections (including tonsillitis and ear infections), and *nasal disuse*, congestion caused by habitual mouth breathing.

Every person (child and adult) lives somewhere on a spectrum that spans from normal/healthy breathing to severe OSA. Because the fragmented breathing progression is sneaky-slow, the changes in your child, are often so subtle that you don't recognize them until there are significant health ramifications. To see a profound example of this, search on YouTube for the gut-wrenching story called "Finding Connor Deegan" by the Foundation for Airway Health.

66

Many of these **behavior issues** are from **sleep deprivation**—the usual sidekick to pediatric airway dysfunction. Because **SLEEP**, both the quality and quantity of it, is so profoundly important to your *child's health*, it deserves a separate chapter (to follow).

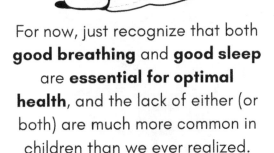

For now, just recognize that both **good breathing** and **good sleep** are **essential for optimal health**, and the lack of either (or both) are much more common in children than we ever realized.

99

In this chapter I'll support you, a Brave Parent, in how to recognize airway disorders and how to advocate for your child when you do. Before delineating the symptoms and physical signs, let's build some understanding of early craniofacial development and how it relates to advantageous breathing.

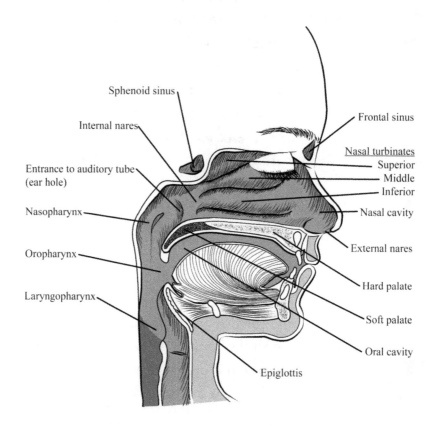

4.1 EARLY DEVELOPMENT OF THE FACE AND BREATHING APPARATUS

Our contemporary ancestors, only 300–500 years ago, had wider noses, straight teeth, and broad, flat palates—in the shape of their flattened tongues. They had, flat-out, bigger mouths complete with plenty of room for their wisdom teeth to erupt and chew.

Deviations from that picture are so common today that we have come to accept them as normal. In fact, the majority of children in industrialized countries have early childhood malocclusion (ECM), typified by abnormal jaw growth, alignment of teeth, and bite. You already know this to be true, judging by how many kids get braces during adolescence these days. But it develops long before puberty, and it has typically delivered health threats far beyond what meets your eye.

There have been many contributing factors to this shift, and they involve early childhood development. Spoiler alert ... these factors are primarily *environmental, not hereditary or evolutionary*. It has to do with post-industrial society's introduction of things like baby bottles, pacifiers, pureed baby foods, and soft processed foods.

Here are the nine associated *oral dysfunctions* that we see as a result:

- Lack of prolonged breastfeeding
- Habitual mouth breathing
- Airway obstruction (including enlargement of tonsils and adenoids)
- Soft tissue restrictions (including lip- and tongue-ties)
- Improper oral resting posture
- Oral habits (like pacifiers, fingers, and thumbs)
- Incorrect swallowing patterns
- Lack of chewing real food (versus swallowing pureed food)
- Uncoordinated, under-functioning, or over-functioning muscles (called oral myofunctional disorder or OMD)

Dr. Kevin Boyd, a pediatric airway expert and consultant to the Sleep Medicine service at Chicago's Lurie Children's Hospital, has really helped me (and my profession) understand the dynamics between dysmorphia (deformity in shape) and dysfunction. I now describe it in this way.

Our *external* human face is intimately connected to the *internal* face by way of the breathing complex. Collectively, we now refer to this internal face as the craniofacial-respiratory complex (CFRC). Beyond breathing, some other survival functions, for which the CFRC is responsible, include verbal and vocal communication, smelling, chewing, and swallowing. For now, let's explore its profound influence on breathing.

Reach up and touch your face, exploring the outside of your lower jaw (mandible). And now your upper jaw (maxilla). You are feeling the contours that shape your external face. But the inside contours of your jawbones (with overlying soft tissues) create a unique space too. That inner "vault" is where your tongue lives. I affectionately refer to it as the "tongue box."

Now feel your nose. It has an outer shape and an inner shape too. The nostril size plays a small part. But more importantly, the internal structure houses a series of labyrinth-like caverns called turbinates that are unique to just you. The patency (openness) of those caverns is a big deal. More on their function and dysfunction to follow.

The nose space and tongue box converge and empty into your pharynx (throat), the larger breathing tube in the back of your nose and mouth. If the pharynx becomes inadequate—either crowded by soft tissue or just too skinny—it will fail to support a healthy breathing experience. The collective silhouette of your craniofacial-respiratory complex truly determines your ability to fuel your body with 24/7 oxygen.

As your child's body grows, if the growth of his jawbones is stunted in comparison, his throat and breathing passageways will be developmentally squashed also. Likewise, when the jawbone growth is stunted, the nose will be narrow, and the nasal passageways will be smaller too.

We must all get better at understanding and identifying the *risk factors (preventive elements)* for this tragedy as well as the best after-the-fact *responses (treatment strategies).*

4.2 MUSCLES ALWAYS WIN

You might still believe that the unique shape of your CFRC must be predicted by a genetic lottery. Not so! While there is clearly a *hereditary* component, the science points instead to the profound *environmental,* face-shaping influences that have an even greater role in modeling the CFRC. These are the early childhood habits of sucking, swallowing, chewing, and resting tongue posture.

To conceptualize this, think of the muscle memory involved in throwing a softball at a target. It's a complex task, but when you copy it successfully enough times that your brain memorizes "your way" of doing it, the repeatable activity becomes somewhat mindless and thus harder to change. Over time, if you've learned to do it harmoniously (from a biomechanical perspective), it can help protect the health of your shoulder, whereas if you learn to do it deleteriously, it can lead to chronic inflammation, injury, and even permanent deformity.

The same is true for the complex tasks of chewing, swallowing, and even "resting" your tongue. But these complicated oral motor patterns are much more significant than ball-throwing because they are repeated in utero and committed to muscle memory through the first years of a child's life—when their bones are completely malleable and rapidly developing. They're also harder to change. The habitual muscle functions of the tongue and face actually *form* the shape of the adult CFRC starting at five weeks in utero and extending to about six years old.

Muscles create competing forces. Imagine a pushing war. The cheek muscles are always pushing *inward*, especially on the upper jawbone. If left to themselves, they would constrict the upper jaw and cause a narrow palate with a high-arched roof.

But along comes the big, strong tongue. Hopefully, it is resting forward and high in the palate, so as it functions, it continually presses the upper jawbone *outward* (both crosswise and forward). Optimally, the shape of the hard palate becomes a mirror image of the top of the tongue: broad and flat!

A roomy tongue box gives the lower jawbone room to expand, so it grows forward and laterally also. Together, these generous, U-shaped arch forms allow for the eruption of well-aligned teeth, a broad smile, and little need for orthodontic treatment.

By now it may seem completely obvious that our ability to form a generous tongue box, uncluttered nose, and spacious throat space sets the foundation for a lifetime of better breathing. Keep this picture of health in your mind's eye as you read further.

4.3 THE MOUTH IS FOR EATING, AND THE NOSE IS FOR BREATHING

Newborns are "obligate nose breathers." That means in order to survive without medical intervention, your baby must be able to *exclusively* use her nose to breathe while simultaneously using her mouth to suck and swallow.

Breathe, suck, swallow! It's miraculous that your brand-new baby arrives knowing how to do *all* of that, as she has been practicing since twelve weeks in utero! But what if your baby is born with an uncoordinated swallowing function? Turns out, if no one intervenes, our swallow has a muscle memory that lasts for life, and if it's dysfunctional it can distort the face, breathing complex, and dental arches. So, if your baby isn't sucking or swallowing correctly, it's up to you to find help.

In today's world, most parents leave the hospital with their newborn without a breathe-suck-swallow evaluation and without any kind of feeding follow-up. This can be a very frustrating, scary, and depressing time for moms especially. Be brave and get help!

Even if you live in a rural setting, a board-certified lactation consultant is worth seeking out. They are skilled at suck therapy, and many of them are good diagnosticians of lip- and tongue-tie. Body-work can be helpful if you consult a skilled pediatric osteopathic manipulation physician or pediatric chiropractor.

You may also want to go beyond suck therapy with analysis of the swallow function including the role of the facial musculature. There is a growing number of feeding specialists in the field of pediatric occupational therapy (OT) or speech language pathology (SLP). Hallie Bulkin, the originator of *Feed the Peds* has trained more than 1,000 OTs and SLPs to help. For a directory of support look at pediatricfeedingtherapist.com.

Between feedings, your baby's resting mouth should look like this: closed lips with the tongue resting up on the palate and the nose doing *all* the inhaling and exhaling. (Check your own mouth while you're reading this. Your healthy resting posture should be the same: lips closed, teeth apart, and your tongue resting high up on your palate.)

Gradually the nose breathing "obligation" subsides, as your baby discovers that the mouth can also be used for breathing. By then, hopefully nose breathing will have become *habitual* rather than *obligatory*. But depending on a multitude of factors we will discuss in some detail, sometimes a child will adopt a mouth-breathing habit instead. It can happen because of a lack of ability to passively close the lips, or from a chronic allergy-driven plugged nose, or even as a result of a bad weeklong cold. Keep a keen eye on that as no good can come from habitual mouth breathing. One 2013 study in the journal *NeuroReport* found that mouth breathing led to OSA, hypertension, and cardiovascular disease in adulthood.

Throughout life, the mouth is perfectly designed for eating, and the nose is perfectly designed for breathing! The nose will warm and humidify the air, filter it from particulate matter, and release nitric oxide gases to help purify it. Nitric oxide production is clearly linked to reduction of inflammation, improved sleep, improved memory, and boosting your child's immune system functions.

"

Between feedings, your baby's resting mouth should look like this: *closed lips* with the **tongue resting up on the palate** and **the nose doing all the inhaling and exhaling**. (Check your own mouth while you're reading this. Your healthy resting posture should be the same: lips closed, teeth apart, and your tongue resting high up on your palate.)

"

The mouth lacks the magical abilities of the nose. Mouth breathing, instead, requires the lymph tissue (tonsils and adenoids) to filter and purify the air. That leads to enlargement of your child's tonsils and adenoids, and as they grow, they begin to crowd the pharynx, causing further *nasal respiratory incompetence*. Do you see how the habit of mouth breathing becomes a vicious cycle?

Because tonsil and adenoid removal is hands down the primary intervention in children with OSA, I will address both separately. But for now, let's get back to early orofacial development.

4.4 BREASTFEEDING AND BOTTLE-FEEDING

I grew up amongst the bottle-fed generations—during a time when pediatricians touted the benefits of formula over breast milk. (If you think that's odd, they also recommended cigarette smoking to relax nervous mothers, adding that smoking resulted in a smaller baby and thus an easier delivery.)

A few decades later, we have 26% of our adult cohort afflicted with obstructive sleep apnea. In a few minutes you'll learn why there is a correlation.

Meanwhile, the word is out. When it comes to breastfeeding, you've noticed universally positive messaging about the psychological benefits of mother-baby bonding and immune-protective benefits of breast milk. Turns out our own nutrient-rich breast milk trumps every factory-made formula ever invented.

But usually overlooked are revelations about the profound impact that breastfeeding has on oral-facial growth and development. The magic is in the sucking!

The complex act of breastfeeding exercises a baby's oral-facial muscles. And poof! Just like in the body, muscles that get repetitive workouts get bigger and stronger. Through breastfeeding, the tongue muscles must work up to sixty times harder to extract milk than it would from a bottle. That means the tongue gets sturdier, and as it assumes its rightful place at the top of the mouth, it has more power to shape the tongue box.

Breastfeeding continues to be developmentally beneficial until babies are weaned onto whole foods. Ancestrally, before we had this universal thwarted oral-facial growth pattern, babies weaned at about three and a half years old. Along with encouragement to nurse longer, I'm fascinated by the movement toward baby-led weaning (BLW) because kids who use their mouths to suck, gnaw, and "chew" foods, even before they have teeth, also help build robust musculature. I discuss BLW in more detail in chapter 3 Digest, section 3.6.

> " But usually **overlooked** are revelations about the profound **impact** that *breastfeeding* has on **oral-facial growth** and development. The magic is in the sucking! "

Conversely, a bottle-fed baby is more likely to develop a lazy tongue that relaxes into a low rest position. A low tongue posture allows the cheek muscles to win the pushing war, pressing inward to narrow the jawbones.

Bottle-feeding carries another developmental risk factor. That tube-shaped, silicone substitute we also call a "nipple" is not nearly as malleable as the real deal. When a baby swallows from a bottle, the tongue pushes up on that nipple from beneath, forcefully pressing that silicone shape into the palate with every suck. The facial muscles take advantage, pressing inward at the same time. The result? The palate becomes further imprinted to mirror the substitute nipple. It will begin looking punched out, resembling the stamp of a little thumb pressed into Play-Doh.

If you choose bottle-feeding, select a slow flow nipple, and don't automatically increase the aperture as the child grows. Just as a breastfed baby never gets to move up a nipple size, bottle-fed babies should build healthy oral musculature as they work harder for more milk. If your baby is destroying the nipple or you're getting frustrated with the time it takes to empty a bottle (more than fifteen or twenty minutes), you can try increasing to a medium flow.

Or better yet, you can go straight to cup-feeding, which helps develop oral motor function without the introduction of a fake nipple. Advanced feeding specialists consider cup-feeding the next best thing to breastfeeding. Does swallowing milk from a cup sound like it would be too difficult for your newborn to learn? It's actually easier and safer and even used for high-risk babies who are born prematurely and not yet able to latch. The WHO recognizes that cup-feeding is used more routinely in developing countries.

4.5 PREMATURE DELIVERY AS AN ADDED RISK

Premature delivery is an added risk factor for difficulty with breastfeeding *and* obstructive sleep apnea. Guilleminault and Huang's research showed that nearly all (82%) infants born before thirty-four weeks gestation have high narrow palates, and most have associated problems with breastfeeding behaviors.

In addition, 82% of preemies (born between twenty-five and thirty-seven weeks of gestation) also had signs of early obstructive sleep apnea. Out of the 9% of preemies that present with a normal-shaped palate, the bottle-feeding they "require" results in high narrow palates and low lazy tongues by six months old.

Get some help with cup-feeding and additional exercises for muscle development from a pediatric expert in OT, SLP, or oral myofunctional therapy.

4.6 PACIFIERS TO THE RESCUE...NOT!

In my early years as a dentist, I recommended pacifiers so a child wouldn't find their thumb. I reasoned that it was easier to squash a pacifier habit than a thumb-sucking habit. We knew they often distorted the mouth, but we had no awareness that it was a setup for airway- and sleep-related breathing disorders for the rest of their lives.

Even though many pediatricians still advise them, we now know they can be a significant culprit in thwarted facial development. With every suck, the tongue pushes up on an artificial rubber bulb, influencing a high arch palate and small nasal space. In addition, the lip guard puts pressure on the dental arches (the bones where the teeth will eventually erupt) back into the mouth ... with every suck. Given the potential for facial, tongue box, and nasal passage deformity, we (pediatric airway professionals) have a lot of work to do to dispel physicians' popular recommendations for pacifier use during naps and nighttime sleep.

Why do many physicians push pacifiers? Pacifier use has been reported to be associated with possible reduced risk of sudden infant death syndrome (SIDS) for infants up to one year old. That's thought to be because the pacifier itself keeps babies from dropping into deeper stages of sleep. This is alarming to me. You will learn in the next chapter (Sleep) why you wouldn't want your child's growing brain to be deprived of deep sleep.

Although we still don't understand what causes SIDS, when you dig into the literature you will find that an increased incidence has more to do with being born premature, mothers who smoke during pregnancy (increasing SIDS risk three times), secondhand smoke (doubling the risk), overheating, tummy sleeping, and sleeping on too-soft surfaces with fluffy blankets or toys.

> Advanced feeding specialists consider *cup-feeding* the next best thing to breastfeeding. Does swallowing milk from a cup sound like it would be too difficult for your newborn to learn? It's actually **easier and safer** and even used for high-risk babies who are born prematurely and not yet able to *latch.*

If you still feel strongly about a pacifier, you should know that the risk of SIDS peaks at two to four months and drops significantly after six months. So, hand them over to the "pacifier fairy" as soon as you feel comfortable.

While it's true that pacifiers *pacify* babies, I find they're more about pacifying the parents.

I love this quote from Dr. Bill Hang, a leading expert in airway orthodontics:

"My wife and I used pacifiers for our kids, like most parents did at that time. Based on current knowledge that pacifiers can push the teeth back in the face, I wish I'd gotten ear plugs for my wife and me rather than use a pacifier for my kids. Live and learn!"

4.7 IDENTIFYING AND CORRECTING LIP-TIES AND TONGUE-TIES

It sucks not to suck! (I often wonder how the word "suck" got such a bad connotation when, for thousands of years, our very survival relied on sucking.)

If your baby has a tongue or an upper lip that is bound too tightly to their mouth, we call those tethered oral tissues (TOTs). Either of these can restrict mobility enough to wreak havoc with baby's ability to latch and to suck. Plus, now that you know how important a high resting tongue posture is for breathing, you appreciate why a newborn with a tongue-tie, binding it to the floor of the mouth, is in trouble from the start.

It's estimated that neonatal ankyloglossia (tongue-tie) commonly affects 20% of babies, so in many cases, even when mom or baby are having grave difficulty latching, it's frequently down-played as "normal" by pediatric health care professionals across the board. Once again, "normal" doesn't mean healthy.

I recently saw a six-week-old baby, Cody, who was literally starving for his mom's breast. He had a (Kotlow Classification) Class IV complete tongue-tie—literally to the tip of his tongue. He could hardly latch, and when he did, he fell off her nipple almost immediately. After performing a laser-assisted tongue and lip release, Cody's mom felt like I had waved a magic wand. Through tears, she reported how terrible she felt that she had waited so long to get to me. She was also angry with Cody's pediatrician, who she'd asked to evaluate her suspicion of tongue-tie on three separate occasions. His response to her was, "Tongue-tie is a trendy, Facebook-driven movement—not a real diagnosis." How very sad!

In fairness to Cody's doc, he is likely an expert on so many health-enhancing subjects, but not this one! If he or she isn't up to date on how to evaluate tongue function, classify lip- or tongue-ties, or on the importance of proper tongue function for effective breathe-suck-swallow development, they should refrain from rendering an opinion. Better to say "I don't know. Let me study this more and get back to you."

The truth is, long before modern medical practices existed, midwives kept one long fingernail to detach a baby's tethered oral tissues at birth. Without her help, a newborn might not survive. This unsophisticated practice dates back to the Middle Ages, but by the eighteenth century there are several sources referencing the need to liberate the tongue to facilitate breastfeeding.

Today it's more customary for the delivering physician or lactation consultant to identify these at birth, but they seem to address only the super obvious ones. Sometimes the doc snips the anterior *frenum* (or *frenulum*) right in the hospital with scissors.

An obvious restriction is usually a front-of-the-tongue-tie (anterior tongue-tie). But docs are starting to recognize a *posterior* tie, too, one that limits the back of your baby's tongue from suctioning up to the palate. Unfortunately, a customary scissor-snip of an anterior tie often results in an incomplete release because a posterior tie requires a little deeper release of the genioglossus muscle, beyond the skin and fascia.

Baby's usual symptoms of a lip- or tongue-tie in a breastfeeding infant include:

- weak latch
- falling asleep while nursing
- reflux
- spitting up
- gassy/bloating/gut pain
- clicking/smacking while eating
- long and frequent nursing needs

Mom's usual sufferings include:

- painful nursing
- cracked, blistered, bleeding nipples
- thrush/mastitis
- inability to empty breasts
- compromised milk supply

To physically evaluate whether your baby has restrictions, use your index finger to sweep side to side under the tongue. If there is a web-like structure or a speed bump, you'll want further evaluation. Do the same to the upper lip. Next, lift the upper lip to the nose and see if it causes blanching (whitening) on the attached gum tissue.

The good news is releasing these tethered tissues is a relatively noninvasive procedure with an extremely low risk of infection. Today, soft tissue lasers make these procedures precise, complete, fast, and relatively painless—and they require no sedation or even local anesthesia. Compared to scissors, laser-assisted tongue release for infants is considered more controlled, less painful, and faster to heal.

As the surgeon, I'm able to elevate the tongue as I release, so I can address the anterior, middle, and posterior elevations. The same goes for the lip. I can lift the restricted lip as I gradually release it.

Each procedure takes about ten to fifteen seconds. And each requires that the parents continue daily stretching of the little wounds for several weeks as they heal. Stretching is important, and I have noticed parents aren't told that if they have a scissor release in the hospital. When we release the string-shaped tissue, it becomes a diamond-shaped wound, and the surface area heals with scar-like cells. Picture a softball diamond sprinkled with grass seed that begins to grow. While it heals, stretching the wound is not about avoiding reattachment, but to maintain the full release, as the scar tissue tries to retract and restrict function.

As a friend to my patients, this experience is amazing. In all my work, I find almost nothing more gratifying than handing a newborn back to mom and witnessing the baby's newfound ability to latch, suck, swallow, and breathe!

If you miss the opportunity for an early release, ties can be addressed any time in life. Unfortunately, they may pose some significant challenges along the way. In addition to constriction of the CFRC, a child can develop speech problems, cervical neck muscle pain, posture abnormalities, temporal mandibular joint (TMJ) pain, chronic headaches, sleep disorders, and associated behavior problems (to be delineated later). To learn more about this for your own tongue restriction, check out TheBreatheInstitute.com where Dr. Soroush Zaghi, an internationally renowned ENT (airway and sleep surgeon), posts much more on *functional frenuloplasty* for adults.

4.8 ASTHMA

Another children's airway disease whose incidence skyrocketed with alarm in the past forty years is *asthma*. The "asthma epidemic" seemed to begin its climb in the early 1980s, rising at an average of 4.3% per year until 2009, when it began to plateau. Today, the CDC estimates that twenty-five million people in the US have asthma and approximately six million of them are children.

In childhood asthma, the lungs and airways become acutely

inflamed when exposed to certain triggers. Allergic (or extrinsic) asthma is triggered by allergens, such as dust mites, pollen, and mold. Nonallergic (or intrinsic) asthma has a range of other physical triggers, including weather conditions, exercise, a respiratory bug like the common cold, and stress. Symptoms can range from being merely bothersome to having a severe attack that chokes out lung function altogether.

> **"**Another children's **airway disease** whose incidence *skyrocketed* with alarm in the past forty years is **asthma**. **"**

For asthmatic children, the ongoing, day-to-day, quality-of-life issues revolve around being tired from lack of sleep, missing school, and the inability to play outside (to avoid allergens) and play sports (to avoid exercise-induced bronchoconstriction). These kiddos often have delayed recovery or bronchitis after a common respiratory infection such as a cold. For some, asthma can cause dangerous attacks, requiring an unexpected visit to the emergency department and potentially hospitalization.

Sadly, this disease does not appear to be curable, and symptoms can continue into adulthood. But today, with the right treatment, you can partner with your child to keep symptoms under control and prevent further damage to growing lungs.

The big question is can you also *prevent* it for your baby? Even though we know the rise in asthma rates is associated with industrialized societies, there is confusion about the root cause elements you would need to control. Still, I can make some guesses based on data correlations. Let's take a look.

For many years there was a mountain of evidence that living in a less hygienic environment with an increased exposure to bugs (bacteria and virus) was associated with a *lower* incidence in asthma. In theory, exposure to certain bugs teaches the immune system not to overreact. This is called the *hygiene hypothesis*, and it's consistent with the rising allergy and autoimmune deficiencies we associate in children who host a deficient germ population (see more about microbiome deficiency in chapter 3 Digest).

Today however, after weighing lots of additional asthma-incidence data from unhygienic cultures around the world, the hygiene hypothesis doesn't hold as much water. In fact, a huge landmark review of all asthma literature showed that fewer than half of all asthma cases are associated with allergy. When separating the allergic and nonallergic asthma cases, there appears to be clusters of different kinds of asthma, each responding to different triggers.

We also believed that early-life infections were protective against asthma, but now they are thought to be a risk.

Sometimes, as in the case of this disease, the more we learn the less we know!

To help unravel the mysteries, the National Institutes of Health (NIH) currently supports a number of asthma research networks. In trying to uncover clusters of different types of asthma, we are hoping to identify their different causes and associated treatment strategies as well.

All of this flux in learning points to your parent role as a health advocate. If you have a child with asthma, make sure you seek the care of an asthma specialist who makes it a hobby to stay up to date on the current literature as it emerges.

For now, here are some best practices to reduce the frequency of asthma attacks:

- Help your child learn to avoid personalized allergens and irritants that trigger his or her asthma symptoms.
- Don't allow adults to smoke or vape around your child. Exposure to tobacco smoke during infancy is a strong risk factor for childhood asthma, as well as a common trigger.
- Help your child stay active with activities they enjoy. As long as your child's asthma is well controlled, regular physical activity can help condition the lungs to work more efficiently.
- Maintain regular medical care with a research-astute physician who listens to you and works well with you as a team. Asthma triggers and symptoms can change over time, so partnering with your child's doctor(s) will help you tweak treatments in order to keep symptoms under control.
- Make your doctor aware of symptoms that indicate your kiddo's asthma might not be under control, such as more frequent need for a quick-relief inhaler.
- Help your child eat whole foods and avoid processed foods in order to reduce inflammation and maintain a healthy weight. Overweight and obesity can worsen asthma symptoms.
- Address heartburn (also called acid reflux or airway reflux). It's generally understood that reflux or severe heartburn can worsen your child's asthma symptoms. He or she might need over-the-counter or prescription medications to control acid reflux in the short run. The proton-pump inhibitors (PPIs) are popular and powerful anti-reflux medications, but they come with a host of long-term complications. The broad-based warnings say not to take for more than two weeks because they interfere with gut absorption of essential nutrients (calcium, magnesium, iron, and vitamin B_{12})

from food. So, in the long run, it's best to identify, from the long list of possibilities, the *root cause* of reflux. If the reflux is from a food sensitivity, obstructive sleep apnea, or obesity, work with your child to identify and improve these so you can help your child de-medicate from PPIs.

When it comes to speculation about prevention strategies, we must acknowledge that asthma disease has skyrocketed in prevalence over the past thirty years. There is something about Westernization that has wreaked havoc with our immune systems. Consider the combination of increased processed foods consumption, out-of-control sugar intake, obesity (an inflammatory condition), lack of microbial diversity in our individual microbiome, and lack of exposure to the earth. The truth is, we don't yet know what that mechanism is, but, as you'll read throughout these chapters, it clearly pays to help your kiddo eat whole foods, get regular exercise, and play outdoors. Sure, sometimes you'll be accused of being old-fashioned, sometimes even mean, but that is the plight of a really brave and loving parent.

4.9 SNORING, NOISY BREATHING, AND MOUTH BREATHING

A flurry of Facebook and YouTube posts suggest that snoring babies are cute and funny. When it comes to your kiddo's health, snoring is neither cute nor funny!

Babies shouldn't snore! Even audible breathing (during wake or sleep) is a smoke signal. Noise should alert you to an airflow limitation or obstruction, a crowded or restricted breathing space.

If your child is mouth breathing or snoring, especially in the absence of respiratory infections or allergies, you'll want to seek a consultation with an *airway-educated* dentist, speech language pathologist, or pediatrician about the possibility of sleep-disordered breathing or obstructive sleep apnea. Recognition and advocacy are hyper-important.

> 66
>
> If your child is **mouth breathing** or **snoring**, especially in the absence of respiratory infections or allergies, you'll want to seek a consultation with an airway-educated dentist, speech-language pathologist, or pediatrician about the possibility of **sleep-disordered breathing** or **obstructive sleep apnea**. Recognition and advocacy are *hyper-important.*
>
> 99

Keep in mind how hungry the developing brain is for oxygen. At birth your baby's brain is only about one-third of its adult size. But by two years old, it's already at 80%! Neurons, at any stage in life, are especially vulnerable to oxygen deprivation, so maintaining optimal airway health in infancy brings with it a big brain advantage.

Let me help you take the blinders off and identify *all* the symptoms, signs, and risk factors of airway disorders and look at strategies to improve breathing. Believe me, it can make a crazy-big difference for a lifetime of your kiddo's health.

4.10 BEHAVIORAL SYMPTOMS OF AIRWAY DISORDERS

Perhaps the most heartbreaking aspects of airway dysfunction are the behavior changes that develop in oxygen-starved, sleep-deprived children. Here are the familiar symptoms:

- Bed-wetting
- Restless or fitful sleep
- Night terrors
- Anxiety
- Learning disabilities
- Aggressive/defiant behavior
- Slowed growth rate or delayed milestones
- Failing memory
- Poor decision-making
- Lack of focus, including a diagnosis of ADD or ADHD
- Depression

By now you might be a bit anxious yourself, picturing your own child, a niece, or nephew, or you may even be identifying some of these red flags in your personal history. If your child has a handful of behavioral symptoms and/or physical signs, it's time to seek professional help. But that poses another problem.

At this time, most medical professionals don't recognize the signs of disordered breathing, or if they do, they underplay them as normal. It's common for docs to recommend a wait-and-watch mode, offering corticosteroid nasal sprays, nonsteroidal anti-inflammatories, and antibiotics galore. It's also common to hear reassurance that a child will "outgrow" airway obstructions eventually as the tonsils begin to shrink, on average around nine years old.

That's not the point. There are about 250 lymph nodes between the collarbones and cheek bones, just to keep these infections in check. So, if a child has a frequent recurrence of whomping infections that necessitate such medication, it means we really haven't addressed the root cause, have we? It pays to look for the signs and symptoms of dysfunctional breathing as well as any physical limitations that might be contributing to that.

> 66
> Recognizing a **breathing dysfunction** problem is tricky because the human body is highly *adaptive.* In other words, we will do anything for *oxygen.* Pay attention to the progression of any number of **physical compensations** such as open-mouth breathing, tooth grinding, strange lower jaw movements, forward-bent head posture, messy chewing, or **strange swallowing patterns**.
> 99

4.11 PHYSICAL SIGNS OF AIRWAY DEFICIENCY

Recognizing a breathing dysfunction problem is tricky because the human body is highly *adaptive*. In other words, we will do anything for oxygen. Pay attention to the progression of any number of physical compensations such as open-mouth breathing, tooth grinding, strange lower jaw movements, forward-bent head posture, messy chewing, or strange swallowing patterns.

Then, put simply, *form follows function.* That means, when the functions of chewing, swallowing, and/or resting tongue posture are deficient, they usually lead to a thwarted growth of the craniofacial-respiratory complex (CFRC) and developmental distortions. The *physical signs* you can look for are:

- crooked teeth
- high-arched palate
- narrow nose
- deviated nasal septum
- underdeveloped upper and lower jawbones
- collapse of the midface (upper lip, nose, and cheekbones)

Optional reading: Some secondary physical signs that deserve deeper explanation are:

- dark circles under the eyes (1)
- eczema (an inflammatory skin rash; this condition also called atopic dermatitis) (2)
- overweight or obesity (3)
- chronic nasal congestion (4)

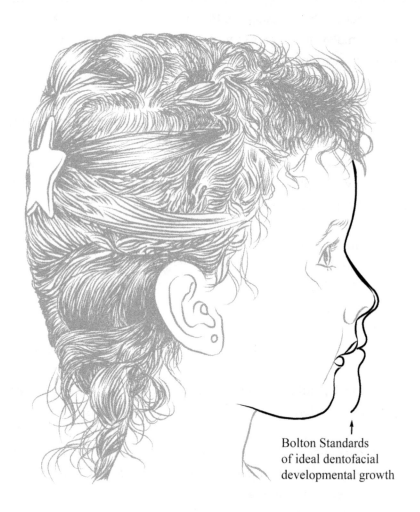

Bolton Standards
of ideal dentofacial
developmental growth

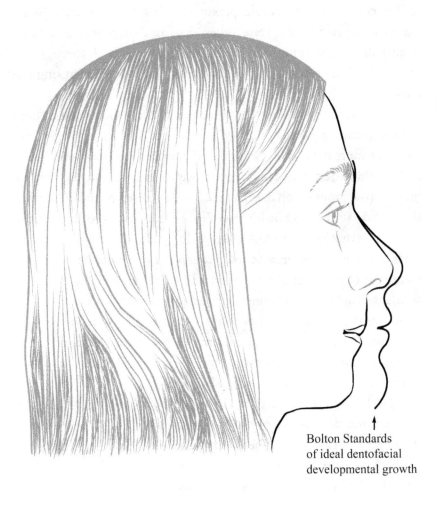

Bolton Standards
of ideal dentofacial
developmental growth

(1) Most parents associate dark circles under the eyes with a tired look. It's actually from retarded growth. Narrowing of the upper jaw also leads to narrowing of the fossae (spaces) behind the jaw. These spaces contain the pterygoid plexus of veins, which receive blood from the inferior orbital vein. When the fossa space is reduced, the plexus shrinks, pushing the darker, venous blood back through the inferior orbital vein. It pools in the skin under the eyes causing the dark circles.

(2) Eczema is now present in about 20% of US children. These kiddos commonly have airway and sleep deficits also. We are awaiting more definitive research to determine the cause-and-effect relationships between persistent airway disorders and the "atopic march" (the progression of eczema, allergic rhinitis (nasal inflammation), and asthma). While it's true that kiddos with eczema can have sleep interruption from the itchy skin itself, there is also some evidence that the eczema actually *causes* the other atopic disorders, including chronic rhinitis (allergic and nonallergic). These can, in turn, interrupt the development of a healthy airway.

Current studies also show that, compared to unafflicted kids, those with eczema have a greater number of sleep problems and a higher measure of sleep-associated oppositional behaviors. Stay tuned for more on these disruptive behaviors.

(3) The associated weight gain appears to have more to do with the resulting sleep deficiency. When your child's sleep is inadequate, the hunger hormones will be disrupted as a result. *Leptin* resistance and the overproduction of *ghrelin* leaves your kiddo just plain hungrier than normal. As a result, airway- and sleep-disordered kids gain more weight than their soundly sleeping peers. (By the way, it's true for adults too!)

(4) Chronic nasal congestion is complicated. There is a tendency for chronic mouth breathing to stimulate what we now call *nasal disuse,* a condition marked by increased mucous production, inflammation of the nasal linings, and a plugged nose. We don't really understand *how* that happens, but that it does happen is predictable.

If you want a dramatic example, read James Nestor's *New York Times* best seller, *Breath: The New Science of a Lost Art.* (Actually, read it anyway. It's riveting and chock-full of compelling revelations on airway health!)

Keep in mind that a plugged nose can be a response to environmental or food allergies too. That poses the question, "What came first—the chicken or the egg?" Did the mouth-breathing habit cause the congestion (the condition of nasal disuse)? Or did the stuffy-nose allergies block the nose and make the mouth-breathing habit a necessity? To answer this for your own child see more about food and environmental allergies in chapter 3 Digest.

4.12 FORMING A NARROW NOSE

Have you heard of people with a deviated septum or nasal blockage who never suffered from a blow to the nose? The plot thickens. It turns out, trauma is not the primary suspect.

You might think the palate belongs to the mouth, but in truth, the roof of the mouth is also the floor of the nose. If it narrows and vaults upward, like a cathedral ceiling, during growth and development, it also reduces your child's nose space. This unwanted thief steals volume from the nasal cavity, and as it squashes the nose, it can physically zigzag (or deviate) the cartilaginous septum, further restricting nasal breathing flow.

From a facial beauty perspective, mouth breathing influences your child's entire face to mature long and narrow. The nose also becomes narrow and sometimes develops a bump on the bridge. That's because the nasal bony spine protrudes as the lower half of the nose (formed by cartilage) slumps down and inward in keeping with the underdeveloped upper jaw.

Dentally, these narrowing arches also result in crowded teeth, and if you're trying to avoid orthodontic treatment, keep reading. We now understand that the majority of these cases are *preventable*.

The first step is to have parents acknowledge when dysfunctional breathing, sleeping, and swallowing patterns emerge.

To quote my colleague Sharon Moore, a brilliant Australian myofunctional therapist and author of the book, *Sleep Wrecked Kids*:

"I often find it is easier for parents to see and understand 'dysfunction' before they can understand 'dysmorphology' (meaning facial structure deficiencies), especially when the child looks like one or both parents."

So, putting aside functional problems, I like to say to parents straight out, "I'm looking at a jaw shape and size that is associated with strong risk factors for disrupted breathing, and right *now* is the perfect age to fix it. Would you like to know how?"

Next, we need to intervene. Let's explore some prevention and treatment strategies to boost airway health such as nasal hygiene, mouth taping, tonsil and adenoid removal, myofunctional therapy, and little-kid orthodontics.

4.13 NASAL HYGIENE

No matter what is causing your child's chronic congestion, it's impossible to restore 24/7 nasal breathing unless you can clear the nasal passages. I recommend regular nasal clearing practice of saline sinus flushes before bed. Sterile saline (salt water), when rinsed through your child's nasal passages, washes away mucous, allergens, and other debris. It also helps moisten the mucous membranes.

It's generally safe, but here are a few important safety instructions to be aware of before you begin.

1. Premix a packet of NeilMed sinus rinse (or other comparable saline product) into distilled water.
2. Stand in the shower, or with your head over the sink, and tilt your head to one side.
3. While relying on your mouth to breath, use a squeeze

bottle or bulb syringe to gently squeeze the saline
solution up into one side of the nose.

4. Allow the solution to pour out your other nostril. Breathe
through your mouth while you're rinsing.

5. Repeat on the opposite side.

6. Try not to let the water go down the back of your throat.
You may need to adjust your head position until you find
the right angle.

7. Finally, gently blow your nose into a tissue when finished
to clear out any mucous.

Young children can learn to do this quite well, but avoid
performing it on your infant. For a demonstration, watch my seven-
year-old friend, Finn. He made a thirty-six-second instructional
video on YouTube. Just search "Finn Nasal Rinse" to watch it with
your kiddo.

If you're looking for an easier approach, try a nasal spray that
contains xylitol (a natural anti-inflammatory agent) with saline,
called Kid's Xlear (pronounced "clear"). One spray before bed and
one first thing in the morning might make all the difference. I
strongly recommend you try both of the above techniques before
resorting to a corticosteroid spray like Flonase.

Another way to help reduce nasal congestion with or without
nasal clearing is *mouth taping* during sleep. Taping is all the rage
with adults these days too. While it may seem like a crazy health fad,
using lightweight, easy-to-remove tape (such as 3M Micropore Tape)
forces nasal breathing and promotes habit formation. It sounds
barbaric, but I assure you it's easily tolerated and safe for any child
who has the ability to pull off the tape if needed. For a few cents
more, try MyoTape—it accomplishes the same thing by gently
surrounding the mouth without covering it completely.

> **"**
>
> No matter what is causing your child's **chronic congestion**, it's impossible to restore 24/7 nasal breathing unless you can clear the nasal passages. I recommend regular *nasal clearing* practice of saline sinus flushes before bed.
>
> Sterile saline (salt water), when rinsed through your child's nasal passages, *washes away* mucous, allergens, and other debris. It also helps moisten the mucous membranes.
>
> **"**

If you notice your kiddo slack-jawed during the day, you can remind her to close her mouth. Rather than sounding like a nag though, try establishing a mutually understood sign language as a gentle reminder. What works well is first making eye contact, then quietly tapping your index finger underneath your own chin as a symbol.

To read more on mouth taping and breathing exercises to support nasal hygiene, check out the book *Close Your Mouth: Buteyko Clinic Handbook for Perfect Health.*

4.14 TONSIL AND ADENOID REMOVAL

The most common physical blockages associated with mouth breathing, SDB, and OSA are enlarged tonsils and adenoids. Most of us give little thought to our tonsils or adenoids. They are little glandular pink lumps in the back of the throat, nose, and tongue. As part of the immune system, they're able to filter the toxins and pathogens we breathe through the air. As you've learned, they become overgrown primarily as a result of mouth breathing.

Some kids get recurring tonsillitis or ear infections, prompting doctors to recommend their removal. But there is another reason for removal. Enlarged tonsils and adenoids, even without chronic infections, often serve as *obstructions* to breathing through the nose.

Abnormally large tonsils or adenoids that obstruct nasal breathing should be removed. According to the National Center for Health Statistics, more than 263,000 children in the US have tonsillectomies each year, and obstructive sleep apnea is the major reason. I'll talk a lot more on pediatric OSA in chapter 5 Sleep. But you should know that tonsils and adenoids (T&A) surgery is considered the first-line treatment strategy for kids over three years old who have a diagnosis of OSA.

Removing the enlarged tonsils and adenoids to unclog the airway helps open the breathing tube, allowing a snoring, mouthbreathing child to get back to quiet, nose breathing. What surgery does *not* help with is getting to the root cause. I always want to know what caused the lymph tissue overgrowth to begin with? And how will we help this child build new muscle habits around a healthy resting tongue posture, swallowing and chewing? So, I've come to recognize that combining surgery with oral myofunctional therapy (OMT) helps to retrain the muscles to better grow/shape the mouth and face.

You might wonder if T&A surgery to open a crowded airway can help intervene *before* a child slips downward to full-blown OSA? The answer is YES, in the short run. It can immediately open nasal passages to support nasal breathing. For long-term results, it works best combined with therapies. Consider OMT, tongue-tie release, and/or early upper jaw expansion (see sections on Oral Myofunctional Therapy and Pediatric Orthodontics to follow).

Not so incidentally, for an obese child with OSA, weight loss is a critical part of the strategy. I'll address more on cause-and-effect relationships of obesity and pediatric OSA in chapter 5 Sleep.

> **66**
>
> Some kids get **recurring tonsillitis** or *ear infections,* prompting doctors to recommend their removal. But there is another reason for removal. **Enlarged tonsils and adenoids**, even without chronic infections, often serve as obstructions to breathing through the nose.
>
> **99**

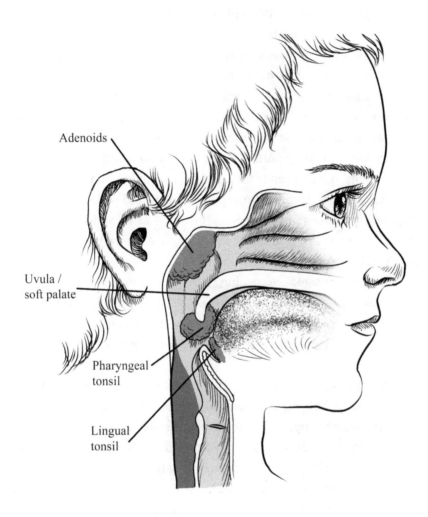

Adenoids

Uvula /
soft palate

Pharyngeal
tonsil

Lingual
tonsil

Without combination therapy, studies reveal that long-term success rates of T&A surgery *alone* to treat or prevent pediatric OSA are poor. That fact makes it difficult to get an ENT to recommend T&A surgery without either a history of recurring infection (tonsillitis) or an OSA diagnosis.

It makes sense because usually, when we're talking about any kind of surgery, less is more. No one wants to risk even the most remote chance of a surgical complication (infection or bleeding) without association-backed endorsement. But in my clinical opinion, equally invasive is the merry-go-round of prescribed corticosteroid nasal sprays, NSAIDs, and/or repeated antibiotic therapies, not to mention long spans of sleep-deprived nights.

It's starting to change. Some pediatricians and pediatric ENTs are responding to the smoke signals—the litany of signs and symptoms that preempt OSA—and advocating for T&A surgery earlier, along with OMT, expansion, and protraction.

Our definitive goal, according to Dr. Christian Guilleminault, the universally most respected expert in pediatric OSA, is *restoration of continuous nasal breathing*. That means that without restoring nasal breathing, we have not addressed the fundamental cause of SDB or OSA.

Pediatric airway leaders in the dental profession have a lot of work to do in helping the medical professions understand how a wait-and-watch approach can have terrible downstream consequences. In the wise words of my trusted pediatric ENT, Dr. Jason Chesney: "There's a lack of understanding from a dental standpoint. If we (the treating physicians) all knew what happens to these kids who mouth breathe but don't yet have frank SDB/OSA or frank indications for adenoid/nasal surgery, we'd be more apt to engage and act."

In the case of an oxygen-deprived or sleep-deprived child with classic symptoms of airway dysfunction, the decision to wait and watch (until it advances to obstructive sleep apnea) instead of building a treatment strategy should NOT be made lightly.

> **66** In the case of an **oxygen-deprived** or **sleep-deprived** child with classic symptoms of **airway dysfunction**, the decision to *wait and watch* (until it advances to obstructive sleep apnea) instead of building a treatment strategy should **NOT** be made lightly. **99**

4.15 MYOFUNCTIONAL THERAPY

There are about fifty-seven oral-facial muscles between your shoulders and your eye sockets that work intimately together every minute of every day. As you've already learned, over-functioning or under-functioning of these muscles are the cause of many abnormalities in breathing, chewing, swallowing, speech, and TMJ function. To address these issues a highly specialized type of therapy was developed called oral myofunctional therapy, or "myo" for short. Myo is a specialized kind of exercise therapy for the face and mouth that teaches children how to re-pattern and reverse harmful habits, and it's accomplished one-on-one with your kiddo and an Orofacial Myofunctional Therapist (OMT) (also known as a Certified Oral Myologist.)

This is not speech, occupational, or physical therapy. It's a specialized kind of individualized exercise therapy, dedicated to help your kiddo repattern harmful oral-facial muscle habits.

Myofunctional therapy can benefit people between two and one hundred years old. (Yes, that means it's helpful for adults who have myofunctional disorders too.) For children, we rely on myo for thumb- and finger-sucking, open-mouth breathing, low resting tongue posture, a tongue-thrust swallowing habit, difficulty swallowing certain textures of foods, messy eating, speech abnormalities, and TMJ dysfunction. We call all these *orofacial myofunctional disorders* (OMD).

The child-therapist relationship begins with a thorough assessment of your kiddo's specific functional habits (both proper and improper) in order to design an individualized improvement plan. Usually in a series of appointments for thirty to forty minutes each, exercises are taught, demonstrated, and assigned for daily practice between visits.

Ingraining proper habits helps drive optimal results. But remember that creating *new muscle memories*—actions that become mindless—requires commitment. It is truly those daily repetitive exercises that help kids convert newly learned patterns into habits.

From an orofacial development perspective, our aim is to achieve proper function as early as possible. But every child has a different timeline for myo-readiness. In my experience, successful one-on-one myo at age two is often wishful thinking. By three or four, many kids have developed a longer attention span, especially for activities that are engaging and interesting, as well as the ability to participate in parent-supervised daily practice.

But even as early as age one or two we can begin with orthotic "trainers," little take-home U-shaped chewing appliances (such as Myo Munchee, Myobrace, or HealthyStart). These are especially good for replacing habits like thumb- and finger-sucking, and they also help to reshape narrow jawbones. Trainers are not available over the counter, which is a good thing, because you will definitely want your airway-astute dentist to be monitoring growth and development.

Successful use of trainers or conventional myofunctional therapy absolutely relies on clear nasal passages. It's impossible to teach nose breathing when the nose is plugged. That means coordinating practice sessions and bedtimes with a quick nasal saline rinse, as discussed above in section 4.13. Then to *maintain* an open airway during sleep, it might mean you'll need to identify and eliminate environmental allergens from your child's bed, such as pets with dander, feather pillows, or dust-laden stuffed animals.

One-on-one myofunctional therapy always aims for improvements in lip seal and lip tone, reliance on nasal breathing, and a more favorable up-and-forward resting tongue position.

The exercises are usually challenging but fun ... actually, borderline silly. My office OMT, Sara, says she and her patient giggle whenever they start a new exercise like playing lip tug-of-war using a button on a string.

When successful, OMT can be miraculous! More detailed goals of therapy are to:

- Restore 24/7 nasal breathing, both in the daytime and nighttime.
- Strengthen and tone the muscles of the tongue, lips, and face.
- Promote ideal tongue rest posture.
- Correct a forward tongue-thrust swallowing pattern.
- Alleviate pain and dysfunction by identifying compensations of the jaw and neck during chewing, talking, and swallowing.
- Prepare school-age, adolescent, and adult patients who are getting ready for jaw expansion, tongue and lip release, significant orthodontic treatment, and/or jaw surgery.

While there's gobs of practical evidence that these exercises work, we continue to need more and better studies to champion lasting results. What the literature is missing are large studies with long-term follow-ups. Also, a recent meta-analysis shows that myofunctional therapists engage in a wide variety of approaches and many different exercises, all aiming at the same objective. More research is necessary to identify and streamline best practices.

To help our professions advance research and treatment strategies, the Academy of Orofacial Myofunctional Therapy (founded by world-recognized OMT thought leaders, Joy Moeller, and her son Marc Moeller) is leading global conferences in collaborative care. Another contemporary research-based treatment organization, The Breathe Institute (directed by a highly respected ENT physician, Dr. Soroush Zaghi) is leading a concerted "myo masterminds" group to help consolidate best OMT practices, while contributing solid, outcome-driven data.

Myo is currently the new buzzword in the fields of dentistry, orthodontics, and otolaryngology (ENT). While orofacial myofunctional disorders have been discussed in the literature for a hundred years, as recently as thirty years ago we only referred for OMT to fix a tongue-thrust that continued to cause the front teeth to splay apart. Now myo is considered almost essential for habit control, infant oral development, support for a tongue-tie release, maintenance for retaining orthodontic outcomes, or in preparation for any kind of jaw surgery.

An important sidenote: As this field continues to emerge, it remains difficult to find a good myofunctional therapist without driving a few hours per visit. The good news is some therapists have figured out how to do great face-to-face therapy using a virtual platform. That's telehealth at its finest hour.

4.16 PEDIATRIC ORTHODONTICS: A NEW FRONTIER

When you think about getting braces for your kiddo, you are probably expecting a referral to an orthodontist during adolescence. Six years old is the earliest an orthodontist might accept new patients, and it's typically for a procedure called rapid palatal expansion (RPE).

While orthodontics refers to moving teeth, rapid palatal expansion, spreading the jigsaw-like "suture" in your upper jawbone, is called dental facial orthopedics, and we are only waiting until six because we thought we had to wait for the first permanent molars to erupt in order to anchor the expander (a turnkey, jaw-widening appliance). But why not before six?

Today's paradigm-challenging question is: Should we be waiting if we recognize a toddler who snores, with retruded jaws, a tonsil-filled jam-packed pharynx, dental crowding, and/or fitful sleep? Are we missing an opportunity to improve a child's physical, mental, metabolic, and neurocognitive developments during their primary years? I think so! And I'm not alone!

From thirty-six years of treating kids, I can assure you that when I see malocclusion in a toddler, it does not resolve itself over time. In fact, it will likely get worse. This is confirmed by the published work of our nation's leading orthodontists, Dr. William Hang, Dr. Marianna Evans, Dr. Barry Raphael, and Dr. Kevin Boyd.

Dr. Bill Hang says: "With forty-nine years of orthodontic experience I frankly get no pleasure out of aligning teeth for adolescents, whose faces are massively recessed from where they might have been had they learned to keep their lips together and become nasal breathers with our early intervention. In my lectures I often refer to straightening teeth in adolescence as 'rearranging the deck chairs on the Titanic.'"

It's difficult for parents to recognize early malocclusion in their kiddo when they are looking at a row of *baby teeth* that are beautifully aligned. Baby teeth, instead, should look like a white picket fence—complete with spaces in between the slats. Straight baby teeth with no spaces in between are a sign that the jawbones are too small to accommodate much larger adult teeth that will be erupting to take their place.

Now I understand that most teenagers who have braces could have benefited from early intervention—expanding and growing bigger arches a few years before the teeth began to erupt.

Because most orthodontists are not accustomed to similar dental orthopedic expansion on kids under six years old, there is a growing need to recruit those who will. This new arena is called pediatric orthodontics. Right now, there is a movement underfoot to establish the International Pediatric Orthodontic Society by Marc Moeller, Director of the Academy of Orofacial Myofunctional Therapy.

If your child is over six, I will talk about a Brave Parent's expectations for the best ortho outcomes in section 7.18 of chapter 7 Chew and Smile.

4.17 AVOIDING BICUSPID EXTRACTION

Traditionally, orthodontists helped align crowded teeth by prescribing the removal of four side teeth (one in every quadrant). From there they created rounded arch forms, while they retracted the front teeth backward, filling the empty spaces. Extracting teeth made their job easier and it resulted in straight teeth, but at what expense? The tongue box just got smaller which crowded the airway space, creating a setup for progressive sleep-related breathing disorders. It also predisposed patients to an increased risk in TMJ (jaw joint) disorders in adulthood.

Two of my colleagues, who practiced separately in the niche of TMJ dysfunction and chronic oral-facial pain, each happened to notice that more than 50% of their chronic pain patients were missing their bicuspids. So, Doctors Michael Gelb and Howie Hindin spearheaded the nonprofits Foundation for Airway Health (FAH) and American Academy of Physiological Medicine & Dentistry (AAPMD) to help turn the trends. Dr. Gelb recalls, "We knew if our professions could treat children with a keen eye on their airway, they would choose expansion and avoid extraction-retraction every time. It was our opportunity to *prevent* the terrible health outcomes we are seeing today." Their book, *GASP*, an Amazon best seller, is not only a good resource for you, but for our dental health professions as well.

4.18 WHO'S HERE TO HELP YOU?

If this chapter leaves you concerned about your own child, you'll need the help of an airway-astute health professional to examine for the oral-facial developmental changes or abnormalities that support a proper diagnosis. They will consider your child's symptoms but also physical contributions to the root cause: tongue position, tongue size, tongue function, tonsils and/or adenoid enlargement, nasal obstruction, deviated septum, and/or turbinate overgrowth.

Evidence-based treatment decisions are sometimes controversial as mounds of research continue to emerge. I will address some of the controversies in the sections that follow.

Meanwhile, the American Dental Association (ADA) now recognizes *dentists* as the primary airway examiners, screeners, and advocates for intervention. It's such a new responsibility that most of my colleagues haven't embraced it yet. Pediatric airway dentists, pediatric dentists, and orthodontists may be hard to find, but they're out there. Be patient while we grow an army of supporters.

In that light, I offer a huge shout-out to my profession to be brave also! We must *all* stay attuned to the literature and adopt new practices as our expectations and evidence-based treatment paradigms are evolving. And while I'm shouting ... attention pediatricians, lactation consultants (IBCLCs), ENTs, allergists, obstetricians, and family docs as well: We need an all-points bulletin to our collaborators across the aisle.

The American Dental Association (ADA) in keeping with the American Academy of Pediatrics (AAP) now recommends that *all children* be screened for snoring and sleep-disordered breathing. The ADA is currently developing a validated screening tool called the Children's General Airway Screening Protocol, or C-GASP for short. It's estimated to debut in 2022.

"

It's difficult for parents to recognize **early malocclusion** in their kiddo when they are looking at a row of baby teeth that are beautifully aligned. *Baby teeth*, instead, should look like a white picket fence—complete with spaces in between the slats. Straight baby teeth with no spaces in between are **a sign that the jawbones are too small** to accommodate much larger *adult teeth* that will be erupting to take their place.

"

We currently use a reliable scale to flush out sleep disorders called the pediatric sleep questionnaire (PSQ), and you can see it for yourself in chapter 5 Sleep.

CONCLUSION

Before I end this chapter, let me ask you this question: Do you see how *all* of this is interconnected? The awesome complexity of the human body can be overwhelming and a lot to digest. Separating the organs and systems of the body first occurred in the late 1700s. It was a modern, man-made construct to help scientists and medical professionals simplify our learning. But you're getting the idea. There is nothing simple here. The body is harmoniously complex, and the role of a Brave Parent, as a health advocate, is to respect just that. When you turn over a big rock and find smaller stones underneath, look under each of those too!

CHAPTER 4 REFERENCES

ADA. (2020). *Sleep apnea (obstructive)*. https://www.ada.org/. Retrieved August 24, 2021, from https://www.ada.org/en/member-center/oral-health-topics/sleep-apnea-obstructive.

Akinbami, L. J., Moorman, J. E., Garbe, P. L., & Sondik, E. J. (2009, March 1). *Status of childhood asthma in the United STATES, 1980–2007*. American Academy of Pediatrics. Retrieved from https://pediatrics.aappublications.org/content/123/Supplement_3/S131.

Angelopoulos, C. (2014). Anatomy of the MAXILLOFACIAL region in the three planes of section. *Dental Clinics of North America, 58*(3), 497–521. https://doi.org/10.1016/j.cden.2014.03.001.

Ballard, O., & Morrow, A. L. (2013). Human milk composition. *Pediatric Clinics of North America, 60*(1), 49–74. https://doi.org/10.1016/j.pcl.2012.10.002.

Basheer, B., Hegde, K. S., Bhat, S. S., Umar, D., & Baroudi, K. (2014). *Influence of mouth breathing on the dentofacial growth of children: A cephalometric study*. Journal of international oral health : JIOH. Retrieved August 29, 2021, from https://pubmed.ncbi.nlm.nih.gov/25628484/.

Boyd, K. L. (2011). Darwinian Dentistry: An Evolutionary Perspective on Malocclusion. *Journal of the American Orthodontic Society, 11*(6), 34–39.

Centers for Disease Control and Prevention. (2011, May 3). *Asthma in the US*. Centers for Disease Control and Prevention. Retrieved August 29, 2021, from https://www.cdc.gov/vitalsigns/asthma/index.html.

Chervin, R. D., Weatherly, R. A., Garetz, S. L., Ruzicka, D. L., Giordani, B. J., Hodges, E. K., Dillon, J. E., & Guire, K. E. (2007). Pediatric sleep questionnaire. *Archives of Otolaryngology–Head & Neck Surgery, 133*(3), 216–222. https://doi.org/10.1001/archotol.133.3.216.

Domany, K. A., Dana, E., Tauman, R., Gut, G., Greenfeld, M., Yakir, B.-E., & Sivan, Y. (2016). Adenoidectomy for obstructive sleep apnea in children. *Journal of Clinical Sleep Medicine, 12*(09), 1285–1291. https://doi.org/10.5664/jcsm.6134.

D'Onofrio, L. (2019). Oral dysfunction as a cause of malocclusion. *Orthodontics & Craniofacial Research, 22*(S1), 43–48. https://doi.org/10.1111/ocr.12277.

Gelb, M., & Hindin, H. (2016). *Gasp airway health: The hidden path to wellness.* CreateSpace Independent Publishing Platform.

Green, S. (2013). Case history: Improved maxillary growth and development following digit sucking elimination and orofacial myofunctional therapy. *International Journal of Orofacial Myology, 39*(1), 45–53. https://doi.org/10.52010/ijom.2013.39.1.5.

Guilleminault, C., Lee, J. H., & Chan, A. (2005). Pediatric obstructive sleep apnea syndrome. *Archives of Pediatrics & Adolescent Medicine, 159*(8), 775. https://doi.org/10.1001/archpedi.159.8.775.

Hanson, M. L., & Cohen, M. S. (1973). Effects of form and function on swallowing and the developing dentition. *American Journal of Orthodontics, 64*(1), 63–82. https://doi.org/10.1016/0002-9416(73)90281-9.

Huang, Y.-S., & Guilleminault, C. (2013). Pediatric obstructive sleep apnea and the critical role of oral-facial growth: Evidences. *Frontiers in Neurology, 3.* https://doi.org/10.3389/fneur.2012.00184.

Kahn, S., Ehrlich, P., Feldman, M., Sapolsky, R., & Wong, S. (2020). The jaw Epidemic: Recognition, Origins, cures, and Prevention. *BioScience, 70*(9), 759–771. https://doi.org/10.1093/biosci/biaa073.

Lumeng, J. C., & Chervin, R. D. (2007, October 8). *Epidemiology of Pediatric Obstructive Sleep Apnea.* Proceedings of the American Thoracic Society. Retrieved August 29, 2021, from https://www.atsjournals.org/doi/full/10.1513/pats.200708-135MG?journalCode=pats.

Marcus, C. L., Moore, R. H., Rosen, C. L., Giordani, B., Garetz, S. L., Taylor, H. G., Mitchell, R. B., Amin, R., Katz, E. S., Arens, R., Paruthi, S., Muzumdar, H., Gozal, D., Thomas, N. H., Ware, J., Beebe, D., Snyder, K., Elden, L., Sprecher, R. C., ... Redline, S. (2013). A randomized trial of adenotonsillectomy for childhood sleep apnea. *New England Journal of Medicine, 368*(25), 2366–2376. https://doi.org/10.1056/nejmoa1215881.

Miller, K. (2020, July 18). *The survival rule of 3 to stay alive in the wild.* theusmarines.com. Retrieved August 29, 2021, from https://theusmarines.com/blog/rule-of-3-survival/.

Moore, S. (2020). *Sleep wrecked kids: Helping parents raise happy, healthy kids, one sleep at a time.* Morgan James Publishing.

Naclerio, R. M., Pinto, J., Assanasen, P., & Baroody, F. M. (2007). Observations on the ability of the nose to warm and humidify inspired air. *Rhinology International Journal, 45*(2), 102–111. Retrieved August 29, 2021, from https://www.rhinologyjournal.com/Rhinology_issues/618.pdf.

Nestor, J. (2020). *Breath: The new science of a lost art.* Riverhead Books, an imprint of Penguin Random House LLC.

Nutten, S. (2015). Atopic dermatitis: Global epidemiology and risk factors. *Annals of Nutrition and Metabolism, 66*(Suppl. 1), 8–16. https://doi.org/10.1159/000370220.

Ratnovsky, A., Carmeli, Y. N., Elad, D., Zaretsky, U., Dollberg, S., & Mandel, D. (2013). Analysis of facial and inspiratory muscles performance during breastfeeding. *Technology and Health Care, 21*(5), 511–520. https://doi.org/10.3233/thc-130749.

Sano, M., Sano, S., Oka, N., Yoshino, K., & Kato, T. (2013). Increased oxygen load in the prefrontal cortex from mouth breathing. *NeuroReport, 24*(17), 935–940. https://doi.org/10.1097/wnr.0000000000000008.

Schneidman, E., Wilson, S., & Erkis, R. (1990). *Two-point rapid palatal EXPANSION: An alternate approach ...* https://www.aapd.org/. Retrieved August 26, 2021, from https://www.aapd.org/globalassets/media/publications/archives/schneidman-12-02.pdf.

Stauffer, J., Okuji, D., Lichty II, G., Bhattacharjee, R., Whyte, F., Miller, D., & Hussain, J. (2018). A review of pediatric obstructive sleep apnea and the role of the dentist. *Journal of Dental Sleep Medicine, 5*(4), 111–130. https://doi.org/10.15331/jdsm.7046.

Tan, H.-L., Kheirandish-Gozal, L., Abel, F., & Gozal, D. (2016). Craniofacial syndromes AND sleep-related breathing disorders. *Sleep Medicine Reviews*, *27*, 74–88. https://doi.org/10.1016/j.smrv.2015.05.010.

Trayhurn, P. (2019). Oxygen—a critical, but overlooked, nutrient. *Frontiers in Nutrition*, *6*. https://doi.org/10.3389/fnut.2019.00010.

Turnbull, K., Reid, G. J., & Morton, J. B. (2013). Behavioral sleep problems and their potential impact on developing executive function in children. *Sleep*, *36*(7), 1077–1084. https://doi.org/10.5665/sleep.2814.

University, S. (2020, July 22). *The toll of shrinking jaws on human health*. Stanford News. Retrieved August 29, 2021, from https://news.stanford.edu/2020/07/21/toll-shrinking-jaws-human-health/.

CHAPTER FIVE

sleep

THE GREATEST UNDERRATED FRONTIER

INTRODUCTION

I f oxygen is our number one nutrient, sleep, it seems to me, should be our number two! It's really not, of course, since water and food are what fuel our cells. But sleep is when all our cells undergo repair and restoration. So, in a nutshell, without adequate sleep, we live in a chronic state of declining health ... and we feel crappy.

In today's world, where sleep deprivation is a pervasive, cultural norm, I can't help but wonder how weighty that is in the cause of our suffering. Our crazy-high rates of lifestyle-related diseases *all* seem to be affected by sleep—both *quality* and *quantity*. Mounds of research show that a chronic lack of sleep, or getting poor quality sleep, increases the risk of cardiovascular disease, cancer, diabetes, obesity, anxiety, depression, and autoimmune disorders.

When I look back at my college years, our mantra was "Sleep is overrated! We'll sleep when we die!" I now realize it should have had a few more words: "We'll sleep when we die, and we'll surely die sooner if we don't sleep." If you've ever pulled an all-nighter studying for a big exam, you might be disappointed to learn, in retro-spect, that when we lose as little as ninety minutes of REM-stage sleep during the night, our cognitive ability drops off a whopping 35% the very next day! Wrap that tip up with a ribbon for a high school grad on their way to college. It might just be the best gradua-tion gift in the bunch. On second thought, why not make it a birthday gift for your six-year-old?

The concept that sleep was overrated began when Thomas Edison invented the light bulb—less than 150 years ago! Edison was a smart dude until it came to his theories on sleep. For some reason he believed that extra sleep made a person "unhealthy and ineffi-cient." He said, "If you put an undeveloped human being into an environment where there is artificial light, he will improve." From a health perspective, he couldn't have been more wrong!

One hundred fifty years of incandescent light is equivalent to the blink of an eye in the history of the human race. In preindustrial days, our sleep rhythms were responsive to daylight and darkness. I guess you could say they still are ... only it's the screen-light, not the daylight, that influences our biological clock these days.

The quality of our sleep is worsening also. We all function some-where on a spectrum from normal/healthy sleep at one end, with snoring and other airflow limitations along the way, then to mild, moderate, and finally severe obstructive sleep apnea (OSA). We progress from cradle to grave, so even healthy aging will move us along the scale, but more important are our lifestyle choices. About 75% of patients with *obesity* have OSA, and that fact would have us think the obesity causes the sleep apnea. The truth is obesity and OSA share a bidirectional relationship, meaning each makes the other worse. That also makes it super hard to correct either one without correcting the other.

66

When I look back at my college years, our mantra was

"Sleep is *overrated!* We'll sleep when we die!"

I now realize it should have had a few more words:

"We'll sleep when we die, and we'll surely die sooner if we *don't sleep.*"

99

Next, if you've read chapter 4 Breathe, you already know that squashing our oral-facial growth and development during our infant and toddler years is mostly not a genetic abnormality but due to lifestyle choices. (Incidentally, if you *haven't* yet read the Breathe chapter, do it now. There is so much overlap between airway health and sleep disorders that you'll rely on those foundational concepts to better understand this chapter on Sleep.)

Your child's *adulthood* healthspan depends on how we approach these issues today. I live in the trenches of advanced airway disorders and it's wretched. It should freak us out that an estimated 26% of Americans have OSA today ... and only 4% have been *diagnosed*. A diagnosis can only be made after undergoing a clinical sleep test called a polysomnogram (PSG) or a home sleep test (HST). So yes, if you google "OSA prevalence," you'll see it's 3–5%. It's the undiagnosed, untreated, ignored OSA that I'm freaked about.

My dad had terrible (undiagnosed) OSA, and his ugly, snoring-sharp-gasping sleep noises rattled my bedroom, which was one floor beneath his. In all fairness, in the 1970s OSA wasn't even talked about. In fact, continuous positive airway pressure (CPAP) treatment wasn't even a brainchild until 1980, when a guy upfitted his vacuum cleaner to help his dog's breathing efforts.

In retrospect, it's no surprise that my dad had six strokes over a period of seven years, considering OSA is a colossal risk factor for stroke. It was heartbreaking to witness. OSA wasn't considered a risk factor then, and it's hardly mentioned now. This is another perfect example of how googled info doesn't tell the whole story. In the US alone, one person dies every thirty-six seconds from a heart attack or stroke, and it's generally pinned on high blood pressure, high cholesterol, diabetes, diet, lack of exercise, or smoking. There are only sparse references to obstructive sleep apnea being at the helm, even though a 2010 study by the National Heart, Lung, and Blood Institute (NHLBI) showed that my dad's OSA *tripled* his stroke risk!

> **66** Your child's **adult healthspan** depends on how we approach these issues today. I live in the trenches of **advanced airway disorders** and it's wretched.
>
> It should freak us out that an estimated **26% of Americans have OSA** today ... and only
>
> **4%**
>
> have been *diagnosed*. **99**

So, c'mon Brave Parents! Let's roll up our sleeves and go to work on *preventing* sleep-disordered breathing (SDB) in your child. And if it's too late for that, preventing its progression to adult OSA! We won't just be fighting for better sleep throughout childhood, but over time, we will be fighting against the sleep-deprivation health threats like weight gain, car accidents (from excessive sleepiness), anxiety, depression, and dementia to name a few. My hope is that between these two chapters (Breathe and Sleep) you'll have enough information to recognize early signs and symptoms in your kiddo and intervene at your earliest opportunity.

In these pages, we will hack into the reasons for our societal sleep deficits more closely—both in terms of *quantity* and *quality* of sleep. This is not intended to be an exhaustive list of all documented sleep disturbances, but I will certainly address the most common causes, effects, prevention strategies, and treatment options.

Fair warning: If there is any chapter that calls for you to be the bravest among all Brave Parents, it's this one. In fact, your perseverance to help your kiddos get *more* (and *better*) sleep, might just get you labeled as the "mean parent." But just remember: Your efforts in raising healthy, happy children, against all odds in today's world, is not a popularity contest. And good sleep ROCKS in the grand scheme of their health!

5.1 A SLEEP-DEPRIVED NATION

How much sleep do we need? More than we're getting. In today's world, half of US children reportedly are not getting enough. Kids learn to devalue sleep from the adults in their lives. The US CDC reports about one-third of adults have a daily sleep debt too.

While it's true that we all have the same twenty-four hours in a day, we don't all *perceive* that we have time for sleep. It's not just that we are working longer hours but that the internet brought with it the availability of round-the-clock entertainment. I have recent hope that our snooze deficit will improve as I see more and more messaging that promotes the health benefits of sleep.

Last week, I had a new patient interview with a thirty-year-old man who suffered from anxiety, depression, addiction, tooth decay, GI disturbances, chronic allergies, and a litany of other autoimmune deficits. He told me that, as a child, he was an excellent student and athlete and that he was really healthy. He said, "I'm here because I need help getting back to being that person—back to being *myself* again."

I asked him to recall when he started to experience his declining health and what he thought was at the root of it all. He said in three simple words: "Lack of sleep!" Then he told me a very sad story.

When he was thirteen, his dad bought him his first video game. It didn't take long before he was obsessed with gaming, and by fourteen, he stayed up all night long to play with his new "friends" (people he would never meet in person). Always tired, he started grabbing two- to three-hour catnaps after school and increasing his caffeine consumption. His grades and sports performance dropped off, but he mustered the energy to hone his gaming ... and his addiction to it.

When I asked him what his parents had to say about his lack of sleep, he replied, "I don't think they ever knew. They were just happy to have me at home, safe and indoors."

Attention all Brave Parents: Pay attention to what your child is doing at night, not just during the day. I know some privacy is important, too, but you still have a responsibility to "see" and protect your child the best you can while they're under your roof. I'll address screen time in the bedroom in a few minutes.

5.2 HOW MUCH SLEEP DO WE NEED?

As we age, our sleep patterns change. But even within an age group, sleep needs vary from kid to kid, even among siblings. You'll have to dial it in on an individual basis while you help them realize the benefits of a personalized bedtime.

For example, my son, Hunter, required more than child-average sleep. And just as the literature suggests, when we found his sweet spot, he was more energetic, sustained a better mood, and absorbed new skills and knowledge more easily. He knew it, too, as we pointed out the *positive* correlation. By middle school, he'd already grown to value his sleep. Even now, at age twenty-seven, I heard him affectionately refer to a personal mood slump as a "no-nap meltdown."

Babies initially sleep as much as seventeen hours per day, which fosters their rapid growth and development (especially of the brain). School-age kids and teens need, on average, about nine and a half hours of sleep. Most adults need seven to nine hours of sleep, but after age sixty, nighttime sleep tends to be shorter, lighter, and interrupted by multiple awakenings. Elderly people are also more likely to take medications that interfere with sleep.

More specifically, the National Sleep Foundation (NSF) recommends that children of different ages get the following amounts of sleep within a twenty-four-hour period:

- newborns (0–3 months): 14–17 hours
- infants (4–11 months): 12–15 hours
- toddlers (1–2 years): 11–14 hours
- preschoolers (3–5 years): 10–13 hours
- school-age children (6–13 years): 9–11 hours
- teenagers (14–17 years): 8–10 hours

Many people feel they can "catch up" on missed sleep during their weekends, but that theory has been debunked. Sleep deprivation fogs your kiddo's brain the very next day. Moreover, chronic sleep deprivation with intermittent attempts to catch up leads to an overarching decline in health—both physical and mental.

FAIR WARNING

66 If there is any chapter that calls for you to be the **bravest** among all *Brave Parents,* it's this one. In fact, your **perseverance** to help your kiddos get more (and better) sleep, might just get you labeled as the "mean parent." But just remember: **Your efforts** in raising healthy, happy children, *against all odds* in today's world, is not a popularity contest. And **good sleep ROCKS** in the grand scheme of their health! 99

5.3 ANATOMY OF SLEEP

Let me start with something you've likely heard about: REM sleep. REM stands for *rapid eye movement* because our eyes literally dart back and forth behind closed eyelids. It's the sleep phase where most of our dreaming takes place, and also where *all* of our skeletal muscles are paralyzed. That's mostly a good thing since it renders us unable to act out our dreams!

There are *three* important non-REM sleep stages also. These take us from wakefulness to REM and from REM back to waking. All three of the non-REM stages take us gradually to a deeper, more relaxed, slower functioning pace. It is actually in the deeper stages of non-REM that help us feel more refreshed and refueled in the morning. During deep relaxation, our body repairs and regrows tissues (including the neurons in our brain), builds bone and muscle, and strengthens our immune system. In fact, it's in the deepest stage (Delta Stage, 3) where the body naturally produces human growth hormone, which helps your kiddo grow and thrive.

If you've ever suffered from the inability to get enough deep sleep, you've surely felt the effects, beyond fatigue—real-life physical and mental deterioration.

Then during REM sleep we get revved. Our brain activity is significantly increased, and so is our breathing rate, heart rate, and blood pressure—to near-waking levels. Not only does a child's time in REM contribute to brain development (especially in infants), but it is also essential for learning, memory, and mood enhancement. Conversely, chronic REM deprivation carries a negative impact on memory, mood, and emotional health throughout our lives. Unfortunately, REM is the phase of sleep most stolen when you have obstructive sleep apnea (OSA).

5.4 WHAT EXACTLY IS OBSTRUCTIVE SLEEP APNEA IN ADULTHOOD?

During REM sleep, when all your skeletal muscles are paralyzed, it is impossible for many people to hold their tongue up and forward, out of the pharynx (throat). Temporarily, that extra pressure creates a collapse, a breathing blockade, and it doesn't take too long before it results in *hypercapnia* (excess carbon dioxide (CO_2) buildup) and *hypoxia* (depletion of oxygen). The cycle is completed when your brain signals for an emergency wake-up call so you can off-load the CO_2 and suck in a breath. We call this an *apneic event.* (*Apnea* in Greek literally means "in want of breath.")

The trouble is, during an apneic event you usually don't even know you're waking up. We measure OSA with a sleep test called a polysomnogram (PSG). These days sleep testing is usually done at home using simple equipment. We count not only *apneas* (stopping breathing for ten seconds or more), but also *hypopneas* (a shallow breath with a decreased airflow) to determine an apnea-hypopnea index (AHI).

If you, as an adult, only experience an apnea (or hypopnea) a few times an hour, your body doesn't seem to suffer noticeable consequences. And since modern medicine hasn't recommended early screening (as we do for some cancers), most people will progress to several events an hour before they garner enough symptoms to report it to a doctor, who orders the sleep study.

That's often too late to avoid brain decline or heart disease. Personally, I think our criteria for diagnosing adult OSA is too lax. If you have an AHI of thirty or above, it's severe. I get that. (Recall that AHI is the average of how many times your body suffers without breath each hour of your sleep.) But what if you have an AHI of fourteen? That's still considered mild OSA—a diagnosis that most patients register as too insignificant to bother with a CPAP. But wait, that means you stopped breathing fourteen times an hour ... or about one hundred times a night! That means one hundred times a night, your brain's oxygen-sensitive neurons were literally starving and suffering. Are you kidding me? There is nothing *mild* about that, in my mind.

Consider this as well. What if, instead of an event being registered as ten seconds without breath, the standard was lowered to nine seconds, or eight, or seven? How high would a person score then? We don't have all the answers, but I promise you this: the scoring standards will look very different a few years from now.

As an adult, if you're fortunate enough to have a bed partner witness you gasping for breath in your sleep, don't blow it off.

> **66** As an adult, if you're fortunate enough to have a **bed partner** witness you *gasping* for breath in your sleep, don't blow it off. **99**

Men have the advantage of erectile dysfunction as an early indicator. Erections are a barometer of cardiovascular health, and an inability to achieve them will generally prompt a guy to talk to his doctor about possible causes. OSA is a well-known cause. Let's face it, erectile dysfunction is *not* what most people associate with the expression "gettin' lucky," but having an early indicator sure beats having a stroke. By the way, it's been hypothesized that the reason women have more strokes and are less likely to recover from them is because they lack such a preemptive indicator.

CPAP is a reliable treatment for OSA, and in some cases an oral appliance that advances the lower jaw forward (in order to open the airway) works well too. The biggest problem with CPAP is patient compliance. Studies show that 30–80% of CPAP wearers keep it on *less than* four hours a night. Machines are getting quieter, and the new masks are amazing, but we have a long way to go for a widely acceptable solution to our growing problem.

ALL of this to ask YOU ... wouldn't it be nice if you could *prevent* adult OSA in your child?

5.5 DOES YOUR CHILD ALREADY HAVE A SLEEP DEFICIT?

If you're not sure your kiddo has a sleep shortfall, I've concentrated the *BEARS Pediatric Sleep Screening Tool* to look at five critical areas: Bedtime problems, Excessive daytime sleepiness, Awakenings at night, Regularity and duration of sleep, and Sleep-related breathing disorders.

See if you answer *yes* to any of the following five questions:

1. Does your child have problems going to sleep or staying asleep?
2. Does your kiddo have excessive daytime sleepiness or a diagnosis of ADD/ADHD?
3. Does your little one experience awakenings during the night (including bed-wetting or night terrors)?
4. Does your child get adequate sleep time?
5. Does your little one demonstrate mouth breathing, snoring or difficulty breathing (such as distorted head or body posture) while sleeping?

If you had even one yes answer, please don't miss a word of this chapter. Your little one's life depends on your knowledge and advocacy.

5.6 OBSTRUCTIVE SLEEP APNEA AND CHILDREN

Twenty percent of children snore, demonstrating airflow limitations. But only 1–3% have true OSA—diagnosed by experiencing one to five apneic events per hour.

We'd obviously like to eliminate *all* airflow limitations before we see this airway collapse, intermittent oxygen starvation, and loss of sleep. Even though there isn't enough published evidence to say that pediatric OSA is a predictor of adult OSA, at this point we see the rate of sleep apnea increase with age, even among kids to tweens and teens.

Just as we see in adults, there is a *spectrum* of sleep-related breathing disorders (SRBDs) in children that you, brave as you are, need to be looking for. To see it, you sometimes have to visit your child's bedroom at night and just watch him sleep.

Pay attention to all sleep-disruptive signs such as snoring, open-mouth breathing, restlessness, and teeth grinding. Take a video on your smart phone to collect "interesting" sleep data. You'll also be able to share it with your airway-astute dentist or physician.

The most common symptoms you might see with sleep-disordered breathing (including OSA) include:

- snoring/noisy breathing
- behavior/mood issues
- ADD/ADHD diagnosis
- marginal academic performance
- bed-wetting
- dark circles under eyes
- allergies or chronic rhinitis

To help you reliably assess your child's risk for sleep-related breathing disorders, google the pediatric sleep questionnaire (PSQ). This risk scale asks you about twenty-two symptoms, including those above, and the cool part is it's a scientifically *validated* questionnaire for kids ages two to eighteen.

When it comes to home sleep testing for kids, replacing overnight in-lab sleep studies, I'm thrilled to report we are getting there! It seems we are in the midst of developing predictable home sleep test options for pediatric OSA including the Nox T3 and SleepImage's sleep ring.

But there are no slam-dunk solutions for treating pediatric obstructive sleep apnea. Once again, it's much better to address the prevention or early progression of sleep-related breathing disorders before it advances to OSA.

As you might remember from chapter 4 Breathe, the first-line treatment for OSA is still considered surgical removal of the tonsils and adenoids. You can expect your kiddo's OSA to improve once the breathing tube is clear, but it's not a concluding resolution. OSA persists after T&A for 13–29% of children with low health risk. In high-risk groups, such as in obese children, the risk of ongoing OSA is up to 75%. You should also be aware that special needs kids have an increased incidence of OSA and advocating for solutions can help them immensely.

CPAP has been historically considered effective OSA treatment for kids, too, and for kids with severe OSA (such as those with syndromes), it can be lifesaving. But the CPAP poses some very significant, negative effects which you'll want to avoid. The face mask has a strap that cinches behind your child's head, creating a continuous compressing force to the midface. At six years old, the human head and face is only at 60% of adult size, and permanently stunting the natural growth of the jawbones can make the structural contribution of your kiddo's OSA even worse.

Sadly, the jaw-advancing oral appliances we use successfully for adult OSA, are *not* suitable for a growing child either.

Our lack of effective solutions has me hyper-focused on what I can do as a dentist, beyond T&A, to improve growth and development. It takes a Brave Parent *and a team* of airway-focused health professionals to arrange early jawbone expansion, a bunch of myofunctional therapy, implementation of an anti-inflammatory diet, allergy control with proper nasal hygiene, and a surgical tongue-tie release, if necessary.

This multidisciplinary approach aims to restore 24/7, uninterrupted nasal breathing. Since these concepts are just beginning to expand among our pediatric health professions, it may indeed require *you* to be the game quarterback *and* the cheerleader as you champion your child. Reread chapter 4 Breathe if you need a refresher.

Here is a hopeful thought. In evaluating pediatric SDB and OSA, I have to remember that children are different from adults. They have muscles that tire more easily, a smaller airway, and less lung capacity. That means the first line of defense is helping them grow a bigger tongue box, as their soft tissues and lungs are developing at the same time. As an airway-focused dentist, it's so fun for me to witness a child become significantly better and quickly blossom. Sometimes we can resolve sleep-related breathing disorders (SRBDs) and even obstructive sleep apnea (OSA) within a few months.

5.7 UPPER AIRWAY RESISTANCE SYNDROME (UARS)

I'd like to familiarize you with another sleep-related breathing disorder that gets little attention in the adult *or* pediatric world today—one I predict will soon become a much bigger player. UARS is hiding from our awareness mostly because, at this point, it's hard to diagnose.

UARS looks something like OSA in its pattern of sleep fragmentation. Also, like OSA, it results from a soft-tissue-crowded breathing tube. The difference is whenever a UARS child stops breathing for a couple seconds, there is a sudden trigger to begin again—and their efforts are indeed successful. That's good because their brain doesn't suffer from high carbon dioxide and low oxygen levels. Despite that,

UARS is a major sleep-stealer. People with upper airway resistance syndrome wake up dead tired. Long-term sleep deprivation from these nagging mini wake-ups (called *microarousals*) can be almost as health-stripping as untreated OSA.

UARS patients will fail a traditional PSG sleep test, and they're often misdiagnosed with simple snoring, or *idiopathic hypersomnia* (a fancy term for excessive daytime sleepiness, and the "idiopathic" part means without a clue as to why). In adults, UARS is treated successfully with CPAP or a lower-jaw-advancing oral appliance. But without a diagnosis, few get treated.

So why is UARS so challenging to diagnose? During a sleep test, without the incidence of arrested breathing for ten seconds or more, and without blood-oxygen dips, the test lacks a true recording of apneas and hypopneas. Your AHI score would look like you're just fine. Do you see how frustrating that is?

So, if you suspect UARS in your child (or you), ask your doc to make a special request for a sleep technician in an overnight sleep lab to continually *watch* your kiddo's breathing—recording each and every respiratory effort-related arousal (RERA) as an event.

Much of this UARS discovery was through the work of a brilliant French physician and sleep medicine researcher, Dr. Christian Guilleminault. He first played a central role in the early discovery of obstructive sleep apnea and helped us appreciate its prevalence in older, overweight people, especially men. Then he discovered that UARS was predominantly affecting younger, fit women, so UARS also became known as the "young, fit female syndrome."

The airway volume of the UARS patient will now be familiar to you: They have an undersized craniofacial-respiratory complex (CFRC) which almost always includes a narrow, high-arched palate, long face with short narrow chin, early dental extractions to remedy crowded teeth, a narrow nose, and jaw joint (TMJ) dysfunction.

> **"**
>
> I'd like to familiarize you with another **sleep-related breathing disorder** that gets little attention in the adult or pediatric world today—one I predict will soon become a much bigger player.
>
> **U.A.R.S.** is hiding from our *awareness* mostly because, it's hard *to diagnose.*
>
> **"**

It was previously thought that UARS was a precursor to obstructive sleep apnea (OSA), and it sometimes is. But UARS is now recognized as an independent condition, crazy harmful in its own right.

My team members and I uncover UARS a lot among my young adult patients, which leads me to believe it's there in teens and young children too. We're tipped off by symptoms of excessive daytime sleepiness, high anxiety, cold extremities, low blood pressure, headaches, irritable bowel syndrome, and early signs of autoimmune disorders such as fibromyalgia and chronic fatigue syndrome.

Our hope for the future is both better diagnostic abilities and better treatment options for children. For now, I continue to predict and preempt UARS by focusing on the same airway-clearing and growth and development strategies we use for OSA. This includes upper jaw expansion and myofunctional therapy beginning as early as age three. Because most orthodontists are unwilling to treat children before the age of six or seven, it opens an opportunity for the airway-astute pediatric and general dentists.

5.8 SRBDS AND BRAIN HEALTH

From birth to age five, a child's brain develops more than any other period in life. At birth, a child's brain is one-fourth to one-third its adult size. Then it grows to 80% within the first two years and 90% by age five. Studies are conclusive that early *neurocognitive* development has a lifelong impact on both your kiddo's intelligence quotient (IQ) and emotional quotient (EQ).

This revelation spotlights the importance of adequate sleep. You see, the brain consists of only 20% neurons. The rest are helper cells, like glial cells and astrocytes—all part of what we call the *glymphatic system*. When we sleep, this army of helper cells kicks into high-gear housekeeping functions in order to clear toxins as well as support, protect, and rebuild neurons. Without deep sleep, they don't get to clean house.

> You see,
> the brain consists of
>
> ## ONLY 20% NEURONS.
>
> The rest are **helper cells**, like glial cells and astrocytes —all part of what we call the **glymphatic system**. When we sleep, this army of helper cells kicks into high-gear housekeeping functions in order to *clear Toxins* as well as support, protect, and **rebuild neurons**. Without **deep sleep**, they don't get to clean house.

Optimizing early brain development was one of the reasons I felt compelled to write this book. My profound respect for brain health is why a "watchful waiting" approach makes me nervous! Pediatric airway problems that cause sleep deficits often get back-burnered because medical professionals have a hunch the kids will outgrow it. Then at six years old, the small tongue box kid is referred to the orthodontist for upper jaw expansion, usually with a directive to fix a dental crossbite, without any acknowledgment of sleep-disordered breathing. Meanwhile, I wonder how much oxygen and restorative sleep that little one's brain has missed during his first six years of life.

I'm passionate about helping with early strategies that include release of tethered tissues for rockin'-good breathe-suck-swallow patterns, habit control for thumb- and finger-sucking, myofunctional therapy, toddler orthodontic/orthopedic intervention, and allergy control.

5.9 OBESITY AND OTHER HEALTH COMPLICATIONS FROM SLEEP DEPRIVATION

At the risk of sounding redundant, I want to list a handful of life-threatening disease states that are directly correlated to chronic sleep deficiency and then talk about obesity in more detail.

In the emotional and cognitive sphere, sleep-worn kids as a whole have more of everything you *don't* want for them: behavioral problems, academic problems, more risk-taking behaviors, anxiety, depression, and poorer decision-making ability in the face of stress.

As for physical and metabolic decline, they might just be headed toward an equally broad range of associated afflictions such as obesity, hypertension, diabetes, heart attack, and stroke.

While each of these cardiovascular and metabolic disturbances are positioned as independent associations to a sleep deficit, it could be that *obesity* alone brings along the other cast of characters. And we have excellent evidence explaining how a person (of any age) might pack on the pounds as a result of sleep deprivation.

At first blush, the sleep-deprivation-to-obesity connection seemed counterintuitive to me. I reasoned that the more hours you spend awake, the more calories you burn. It's just the opposite, actually. Sleep restriction affects our energy balance by decreasing our energy output during exercise as well as our resting metabolic rate (our calorie burn rate during non-exercise time).

And there's an even more critical reason for the shift in metabolism. Sleep loss tips the balance scale on two significant hunger hormones.

Leptin is one your fat cells normally generate in response to eating. It sends signals to tell your brain you're no longer hungry. Lack of sleep mutes this signal, causing a condition called leptin resistance. It keeps your appetite overstimulated. (By the way, sugar does the same thing, as you read about in chapter 3 Digest.)

Next, *ghrelin* is produced in the stomach—it's what makes your tummy growl when you're hungry—and it triggers the brain to stimulate your appetite. Sleep loss drives ghrelin production, and you flat-out eat more.

To me, it sounds like a really bad dream where you wake up sluggish with an insatiable food craving. Meanwhile, your brain fatigue mutes any remnant of discipline to steer clear of chips and chocolate cake—and trust me, those are *not* habits you want your kids latching onto.

5.10 CAFFEINE-CRAZED NATION

Caffeine is our favorite pick-me-up drug of choice. Seventy-three percent of US kids today consume caffeine daily, according to a 2014 survey published in *Pediatrics*, the peer-reviewed journal of the American Academy of Pediatrics (AAP). Shocking as that may be, it's no surprise that daily caffeine intake rises to 92% among college students. High school and college kids are drinking more coffee and energy drinks, whereas school-age kids are getting it primarily in sugar-sweetened soda. All age groups are in the midst of a rising tendency to choose caffeined-up energy drinks over soda. (More on this in chapter 2 Drink.)

Caffeine seems to be ladled into everything these days, and it's touted as a performance drug. It works by temporarily stimulating brain function by blocking the receptors to our natural sleeping hormone, *adenosine*.

The negative side effects are many. Caffeine consumption can lead to insomnia, nervousness and restlessness, stomach irritation, nausea, and increased heart rate and respiration. Larger doses might cause headache, anxiety, agitation, and chest pain.

Think about this calamity for a minute. Children of today are *habitually* consuming an addictive, pharmacological stimulant that increases stress hormones and brain activity throughout every day! No wonder it can cause anxiety and restlessness. I'm catastrophizing this at the risk of sounding like a caffeine-demonizing crazy lady because I believe we've simply forgotten that there's another remarkable remedy to our overarching sluggishness, and it's called (drumroll please) ... SLEEP!

While drug stimulants, like caffeine, can give you some pep, they absolutely cannot override your body's profound need for real sleep. And they often make it harder to fall asleep at night, which further robs you of sleep. Then you wake up tired and want even more caffeine. That's called a *vicious cycle*. You get the point.

5.11 STIMULANTS: THE PHARMACOLOGICAL "RESOLUTION" FOR ADHD

Some kids are getting jazzed by a bigger thunderbolt than caffeine though. Amphetamines are all the rage in today's world. (Amphetamines used to be called "speed"—a highly addictive, recreational drug that has been around for my lifetime and then some.)

" What if your child's ADHD
is a misdiagnosis?

... and those **fidgety**, mentally
fatigued, impulsive behaviors
are really a result of a **sleep
disturbance**, perhaps from
sleep-disordered breathing
(**SDB**) or obstructive
sleep apnea (**OSA**)?

Sadly, this accounts for an estimated
37% of misdiagnosed ADHD.

... Should these kids be
downing a stimulant that
further interrupts their ability to
get a *good night's sleep*?
I should think not. **"**

Among US high school and college kids, Adderall (and others) has been popularized as "study drugs" because it claims to calm their brains and help them focus. The data shows as few as 7% and as many as 33% of college students abuse them, varying by individual campus. These are prescription drugs, prescribed for ADHD, but sold illicitly and used as study drugs.

Even in 2011, I remember Hunter asking me if I thought it would be okay for him to take Adderall before sitting for his precollege SAT exam. It seemed that all his friends were hyping the idea. My answer was simple. "Even if this drug should boost your performance, don't you want to get into a college that is a good fit for your *real* brainpower, not your *artificially enhanced* one?"

By the way, while Adderall might help unfocused kids pay attention, very few direct cognitive improvements have been shown in the research.

But despite the warnings about their long-term side effects, this stimulant craze is here to stay. Over the past decade the manufacturing of prescription stimulants has increased by a whopping *nine million percent*! To me, that's frightening!

It's because today, our ADHD kiddos (oh, plus tweens, teens, and adults too) are given scripts to take amphetamines like they were popcorn! Docs choose between two basic meds: *amphetamine* (the active ingredient in Adderall, Vyvanse, and Dexedrine) and *methylphenidate* (the active ingredient in Ritalin, Concerta, and Focalin).

Doesn't it sound counterintuitive to give our most "wired" kids these speed-up drugs? But it seems to help them focus their thoughts by increasing dopamine levels in the brain. (Dopamine is a neurotransmitter associated with pleasure, attention, motivation, and movement.)

Except here's a major conundrum: What if your child's ADHD is a misdiagnosis ... and those fidgety, mentally fatigued, impulsive behaviors are really a result of a sleep disturbance, perhaps from sleep-disordered breathing (SDB) or obstructive sleep apnea (OSA)? Sadly, this accounts for an estimated 37% of misdiagnosed ADHD.

Should *these* kids be downing a stimulant that further interrupts their ability to get a good night's sleep? I should think not.

Pay attention Brave Parents. The four most common sleep disturbances associated with ADHD sound *exactly* like those associated with sleep-disordered breathing (SDB): difficulty falling asleep, restless sleep, difficulty waking up, and daytime sleepiness. So, *before* you accept an ADHD diagnosis and make a decision to rely on a prescription stimulant, make sure you have your beloved child evaluated for a sleep-related airway dysfunction.

The science supports my recommendation. The conclusion of a large 2014 meta-analysis on the relationship between ADHD symptoms and SDB states clearly that "patients with ADHD symptomatology should receive SDB screening," and "treatment of comorbid SDB should be considered before medicating the ADHD symptoms, if present."

Here's a scary factoid I stumbled upon in my research: Children and teenagers who have been diagnosed with ADHD are also at higher risk for drug and alcohol abuse, regardless of the medication used. The question of the day is, does the ADHD predispose a child to the risk of drug and alcohol abuse? Or could it be because of their early dependency on a mind-altering drug used to treat the ADHD? We don't yet know the answer to this or many other dilemmas like this one.

I'm also curious about some in-process studies exploring how iron deficiency may contribute to the severity of ADHD symptoms and restless legs syndrome (RLS). It's up to all of us to keep asking questions. It is indeed our curiosity that drives new and better research.

5.12 SLEEP HYGIENE

It's time to look beyond sleep-related breathing disorders (SRBDs) and dive into a collection of habits and behaviors known to promote good sleep. Collectively, these are referred to as *sleep hygiene*. But read these at your own risk. Whereas advocating for help with your child's airway deficit can elevate you to hero status, getting disciplined about adopting new sleep hygiene routines at home can turn you into an antihero lickety-split.

(My dear Brave Parent, this is a fitting time to remind you that your child might soon be confused and resort to calling you the "mean parent" by accident. Don't worry ... your treasured kiddo *will* thank you ... later! XO, Dr. Susan)

Because this list of should-dos is long, you might have better success by being up front in describing to your kids the grand scheme of things—your end goals—and then revamping sleep habits one bold behavior change at a time.

- **Get strict about bedroom time.** Notice I just called it *bedroom time*, not bedtime. "Love and Logic" parenting guru, Jim Fay, explained to me years ago that no human (or animal for that matter) has the ability to sleep on command. Our job is to create a space and time that is conducive to good snoozing ... a sleeping sanctuary, so to speak. Create it together and encourage them to enjoy it. I'll describe more about ideal bedroom conditions in a minute.

Sticking to an established bedroom time is a big deal. My now-adult son, Hunter, recently recounted what a drag it sometimes was to have a strictly enforced bedroom time during his childhood—especially when it was still daylight at 8:30ish in the summertime. FOMO, fear of missing out, is a real thing ... even for grown-ups. Ask me how I know. LOL

I was generally more lenient than his dad, so Dan got the bad guy rap. Now at twenty-seven, Hunter is grateful for his dad's persistence —he truly remembers his dad's voice as one of advocacy, not nagging. As an adult, Hunter continues to protect his valued sleep, knowing just how sensitive his brain and body are to a lack of it.

Incidentally, we tried to keep the same bedroom time on weekends as on school nights. It's evidenced that altering it during the weekend makes it more difficult for kids to maintain their normal weekday schedules. Don't be afraid to vary bedroom times even among your own children, depending on their particular needs. For example, between my two nephews, only three years apart in age, Michael (the oldest) required more sleep than his brother (and he still does at thirty-one). If they went to sleep at the same time, Daniel's feet would inevitably hit the ground in a full-on run at 6:00 a.m., disrupting their snoozing household.

Turning in earlier shouldn't be seen as a punishment if you continue to highlight how important it is to find beauty in fulfilling our individual needs.

- **Design some pre-bedroom-time routines.** Repeatable winding-down behaviors signal that it's time to relax and prepare for sleep. Make it simple, tailored to your child's personality, and about twenty minutes in duration. This can include some low-key activities like puzzles, reading together, gentle back rubs, sharing daily gratitudes, or prayer.
- **Waking up should be a natural process too.** In today's world we tend to forget that we're naturally wired to fall asleep when we're tired and to wake up when we're rested. Once again, industrialization prompted this shift. People in the 1800s started staying up late, by lamplight, and they started needing a forced wake-up call in order to show up on time for work. That paved the way toward

the adjustable alarm clock, patented in 1847—just a
moment ago in our human history.

That's not the way it's supposed to work. If your kiddo relies on
an alarm clock (or an obliging parent) in order to get up and moving
in the morning, she probably didn't get enough sleep that night.
Presuming you've already ruled out a sleep disorder, it's a good idea
to ratchet back her bedroom time, little by little, until you experience
a cheerful, voluntary wake-up, without prompting.

And while we're on alarm clocks, definitely lose the snooze function. Here's why:

When you wake with an ALARM, you experience a sudden jolt
from a deep sleep. That experience epitomizes the dictionary definition of the word alarm: to cause (someone) to feel frightened,
disturbed or in danger. Your alarm clock is a shocker—it stimulates a
sympathetic nervous reaction from an adrenaline rush. That fight-
or-flight response can be a lifesaving response to a catastrophe during our waking hours, but it's certainly not a healthy way to
wake up.

When you push the snooze button and drift back to sleep, your
heart rate and respiration start to settle back down, only to repeat
the alarm in a few more minutes.

- **Establish a screen time curfew.** Unfortunately, looking
  at phones, tablets, and TV before bed is not at all
  conducive to healthy sleep. First, screens emit a type of
  blue light that suppresses a natural sleep hormone called
  melatonin. Kid-brains are particularly susceptible to the
  biologic signal that it's daylight—time to wake up.

So be ultra-brave and lay down a hard "NO" rule about electronic
devices in the bedroom. And while you're at it, say NO to any screen
time within one hour of bedtime. You may want to consult

the "Family Media Plan" created by the American Academy of Pediatrics.

- **Pay attention to light levels.** Start dimming the lights in your home as bedtime draws near. Installing dimmers on your light switches will help you better mimic outdoor light after sunset. Keep your child's room as dark as possible and avoid introducing night lights in your child's immediate sleeping space.
- **Make sure your kids are getting enough exercise.** They need at least an hour a day of vigorous play. It doesn't take validated research to know exercise is conducive to good sleep. What do we say while we're watching our kids play hard? "Wow! They'll be sleeping hard tonight!" The studies prove it, nonetheless, telling us that physical activity every day helps people of all ages fall asleep faster and stay asleep longer.

Just make sure your kiddos wind down and avoid spirited activity within two hours of bedtime or they can feel wound up and find it harder to fall asleep.

Because exercise is such an important element of a healthy lifestyle, it has its own Brave Parent chapter 8 Move.

- **Avoid scary or violent content during bedroom time.** That means no scary or violent movies, TV, video games, books, or even ghost stories in the evening. Gore creates worry for kids—it has become a common reason they can't sleep. Some experts will advise you to save the spooky stuff for the daylight hours. I say, avoid it altogether. After all, there's plenty of time in life to grapple with the dark side of human nature. Relish your children's innocence while you can.
- **Nix the caffeine!** This should be a no-brainer now that

we've covered it in detail. Even small amounts of caffeine can have a big impact in a little person. I suggest avoiding it altogether, but if you let them partake, insist they avoid it, even in chocolate, for six hours prior to bedtime.

- **Chill out your home at bedtime.** In order for any of us to sleep well, our core temperature needs to dip. Ideally, we should set our nighttime thermostat about sixty-five degrees. Healthy, full-term babies, lightly dressed, are comfortable between sixty-five and seventy-two degrees. For babies, sleeping in a room that's too warm is associated with a higher incidence of SIDS. If you have a preterm baby, talk to your doctor about the best sleeping temp for the time being.
- **Make bedroom time quiet time.** Your kiddo's sleep quality is affected by even mild sound disturbances. Little sounds won't wake the sleeper to consciousness, but they can still rob her of deep, restorative sleep. If your home has street noise, consider noise-blocking curtains or using a white noise machine to drown it out. And if you snore, don't consider bed-sharing or even bedroom-sharing.

Speaking of bed-sharing, co-sleeping has become quite a controversial subject. On one hand, the American Academy of Pediatrics (AAP) advises that parents should never let their infant sleep in bed with them. There is valid research linking co-sleeping with an increased risk of death from suffocation and SIDS. So, the AAP promotes room-sharing, just not bed-sharing.

On the other hand, there is a lot of support for the thought that co-sleeping stimulates enhanced parent bonding and promotes security. Bed-sharing makes nighttime feedings much more convenient and generally results in more sleep time for mom and baby.

But many people tout the opposite too. Toddlers who are restless co-sleepers (a symptom of a possible airway disorder) can rob parents of good sleep, just as a snoring parent (or two) can repeat-edly rouse a baby from his critically necessary deep sleep.

If you've decided to co-sleep with your little one, read more about how to prepare your bed to share it safely by visiting the La Leche League website.

- **Attend to bedroom time worry.** As you already know, childhood anxiety is steadily rising, and bedroom time might intermittently become worry time. Rather than getting in the habit of lying with your child until she's asleep, try helping her learn to manage her own concerns. Consider setting aside another worry time during an earlier part of the day where you hear their concerns and teach them how to cope.

Bedroom time is a good time for regular practices of *mindful meditation* and *breath work*. Read more about mindfulness-based healing practices in chapter 6 Feel and Think.

If anxiety-driven sleeplessness persists, especially in response to a traumatic event, you will want to consult professional help.

CONCLUSION

Whew! That's a lot on sleep. Are you still awake? Since you are the kind of parent who puts your kid first (otherwise you wouldn't be reading this book), I hope you also understand the importance of *your own* good sleep. Do you also remember what the flight atten-dant announces during the preflight safety rules? "Should the cabin lose pressure, oxygen masks will drop from the overhead area. Please place the mask *on your own* mouth and nose *before assisting others.*" Sleep long and sleep well tonight, my dedicated Brave Parent!

CHAPTER 5 REFERENCES

Aberg, S. E. (2021, January 28). *"Study drug" abuse by college Students: What you need to know.* National Center for Health Research. Retrieved August 29, 2021, from https://www.center4research.org/study-drug-abuse-college-students/.

Alhola, P., & Polo-Kantola, P. (2007). *Sleep deprivation: Impact on cognitive performance.* Neuropsychiatric disease and treatment. Retrieved August 29, 2021, from https://www.ncbi.nlm.nih.gov/pmc/articles/PMC2656292/.

ASA Authors & Reviewers Sleep Physician at American Sleep Association Reviewers and Writers Board-certified sleep M.D. physicians. (2021, July 27). *What is sleep & Why is it important for health?* American Sleep Association. Retrieved August 29, 2021, from https://www.sleepassociation.org/about-sleep/what-is-sleep/.

Bassetti, C. L., Pelayo, R., & Guilleminault, C. (2005). Idiopathic hypersomnia. *Principles and Practice of Sleep Medicine,* 791–800. https://doi.org/10.1016/b0-72-160797-7/50073-2.

CDC. (2020, September 8). *Heart disease facts.* Centers for Disease Control and Prevention. Retrieved August 29, 2021, from https://www.cdc.gov/heartdisease/facts.htm.

Chan, J., Edman, J. C., & Koltai, P. J. (2004, March 1). *Obstructive sleep apnea in children.* American Family Physician. Retrieved August 29, 2021, from https://www.aafp.org/afp/2004/0301/p1147.html.

Chervin, R. D., Hedger, K., Dillon, J. E., & Pituch, K. J. (2000). Pediatric sleep Questionnaire (psq): Validity and reliability of scales FOR Sleep-disordered Breathing, snoring, sleepiness, and behavioral problems. *Sleep Medicine, 1*(1), 21–32. https://doi.org/10.1016/s1389-9457(99)00009-x.

Colten, H. R., & Altevogt, B. M. (2006). *Sleep disorders and sleep deprivation: An unmet public health problem.* Institute of Medicine.

Galgani, J., & Ravussin, E. (2008). Energy metabolism, fuel selection and body weight regulation. *International Journal of Obesity, 32*(S7). https://doi.org/10.1038/ijo.2008.246.

Gelb, M., & Hindin, H. (2016). *Gasp airway health: The hidden path to wellness.* CreateSpace Independent Publishing Platform.

Goyal, M., & Johnson, J. (2017). *Obstructive sleep apnea diagnosis and management.* Missouri medicine. Retrieved August 29, 2021, from https://www.ncbi.nlm.nih.gov/pmc/articles/PMC6140019/.

Gozal, D., Tan, H.-L., & Kheirandish-Gozal, L. (2020, March 24). *Treatment of obstructive sleep apnea in children: Handling the unknown with precision.* Journal of clinical medicine. Retrieved August 29, 2021, from https://www.ncbi.nlm.nih.gov/pmc/articles/PMC7141493/.

Hardy, J. (2021, January 6). *Sleeping in: A short history on sleep before the industrial revolution.* History Cooperative. Retrieved August 29, 2021, from https://historycooperative.org/a-short-history-on-sleep-before-the-industrial-revolution/.

Havard medical school. (n.d.). *Understanding the results.* Understanding the Results | Sleep Apnea. Retrieved August 29, 2021, from https://healthysleep.med.harvard.edu/sleep-apnea/diagnosing-osa/understanding-results.

Hirshkowitz, M., Whiton, K., Albert, S. M., Alessi, C., Bruni, O., DonCarlos, L., Hazen, N., Herman, J., Katz, E. S., Kheirandish-Gozal, L., Neubauer, D. N., O'Donnell, A. E., Ohayon, M., Peever, J., Rawding, R., Sachdeva, R. C., Setters, B., Vitiello, M. V., Ware, J. C., & Adams Hillard, P. J. (2015). National sleep Foundation's sleep time duration recommendations: Methodology and Results summary. *Sleep Health,* *1*(1), 40–43. https://doi.org/10.1016/j.sleh.2014.12.010.

Huon, L.-K., & Guilleminault, C. (2020). Signs and symptoms of obstructive sleep apnea and upper airway resistance syndrome. *Sleep Apnea and Snoring,* 6–12. https://doi.org/10.1016/b978-0-323-44339-5.00002-x.

Jehan, S., Farag, M., Zizi, F., Pandi-Perumal, S. R., Chung, A., Truong, A., Jean-Louis, G., Tello, D., & McFarlane, S. L. (2018). *Obstructive sleep apnea and stroke.* Sleep medicine and disorders : international journal. Retrieved August 29, 2021, from https://www.ncbi.nlm.nih.gov/pmc/articles/PMC6340906/.

Kirby, T. (2011). Colin Sullivan: Inventive pioneer of sleep medicine. *The Lancet, 377*(9776), 1485–6736. https://doi.org/10.1016/s0140-6736(11)60589-8.

Li, W.-C., Hsiao, K.-Y., Chen, I.-C., Chang, Y.-C., Wang, S.-H., & Wu, K.-H. (2011). Serum leptin is associated with cardiometabolic risk and predicts metabolic syndrome in Taiwanese adults. *Cardiovascular Diabetology, 10*(1), 36. https://doi.org/10.1186/1475-2840-10-36.

Lumeng, J. C., & Chervin, R. D. (2008). Epidemiology of pediatric obstructive sleep apnea. *Proceedings of the American Thoracic Society, 5*(2), 242–252. https://doi.org/10.1513/pats.200708-135mg.

Mayo Clinic Staff. (2020, October 3). *Pediatric obstructive sleep apnea.* Mayo Clinic. Retrieved August 29, 2021, from https://www.mayoclinic.org/diseases-conditions/pediatric-sleep-apnea/symptoms-causes/syc-20376196.

Meredith, H. V. (1953, October 1). *GROWTH in head WIDTH during the first twelve years of life.* American Academy of Pediatrics. Retrieved August 29, 2021, from https://pediatrics.aappublications.org/content/12/4/411.

Moore, S. (2020). *Sleep wrecked kids: Helping parents raise happy, Healthy Kids, one sleep at a time.* Morgan James Publishing.

Munafo, D. (2020, July 28). *The connection between sleep and obesity.* BetterNight Solutions. Retrieved August 29, 2021, from https://www.betternightsolutions.com/news/obesity-and-sleep-apnea.

National Heart Lung and Blood Institute. (n.d.). *Sleep deprivation and deficiency.* National Heart Lung and Blood Institute. Retrieved August 29, 2021, from https://www.nhlbi.nih.gov/health-topics/sleep-deprivation-and-deficiency.

Nestor, J. (2020). *Breath: The new science of a lost art.* Riverhead Books, an imprint of Penguin Random House LLC.

Others, R. D. M. E. and, & Ayas, B. M. and N. T. (2016, September 8). *CPAP in obstructive sleep Apnea: Nejm.* New England Journal of

Medicine. Retrieved August 29, 2021, from https://www.nejm.org/doi/full/10.1056/NEJMc1613219.

Paruthi, S., Brooks, L. J., D'Ambrosio, C., Hall, W. A., Kotagal, S., Lloyd, R. M., Malow, B. A., Maski, K., Nichols, C., Quan, S. F., Rosen, C. L., Troester, M. M., & Wise, M. S. (2016). Recommended amount of sleep for pediatric Populations: A consensus statement of the American Academy of sleep medicine. *Journal of Clinical Sleep Medicine*, *12*(06), 785–786. https://doi.org/10.5664/jcsm.5866.

Peever, J., & Fuller, P. M. (2017). The biology of REM sleep. *Current Biology*, *27*(22), R1237–R1248. https://doi.org/10.1016/j.cub.2017.10.026.

Peppard, P. E., Young, T., Barnet, J. H., Palta, M., Hagen, E. W., & Hla, K. M. (2013). Increased prevalence of sleep-disordered breathing in adults. *American Journal of Epidemiology*, *177*(9), 1006–1014. https://doi.org/10.1093/aje/kws342.

Pietrangelo, A. (2018, September 29). *The effects of caffeine on your body*. Healthline. Retrieved August 29, 2021, from https://www.healthline.com/health/caffeine-effects-on-body#:~:text=Caffeine%20consumption%20is%20generally%20considered,individuals%20(54%2C%2055%20).

Quan, S. F., Howard, B. V., Iber, C., Kiley, J. P., Nieto, F. J., O'Connor, G. T., Rapoport, D. M., Redline, S., Robbins, J., Samet, J. M., & Wahl, P. W. (1997, December). *The sleep heart health study: Design, rationale, and methods*. Sleep. Retrieved August 29, 2021, from https://pubmed.ncbi.nlm.nih.gov/9493915/.

Ronald D. Chervin, M. D. (2007, March 1). *Pediatric sleep questionnaire*. Archives of Otolaryngology–Head & Neck Surgery. Retrieved August 29, 2021, from https://jamanetwork.com/journals/jamaotolaryngology/fullarticle/484678.

SCHMID, S. E. B. A. S. T. I. A. N. M., HALLSCHMID, M. A. N. F. R. E. D., JAUCH-CHARA, K. A. M. I. L. A., BORN, J. A. N., & SCHULTES, B. E. R. N. D. (2008). A single night of sleep deprivation increases Ghrelin levels and feelings of hunger in normal-weight healthy men. *Journal of Sleep Research*, *17*(3), 331–334. https://doi.org/10.1111/j.1365-2869.2008.00662.x.

Sedky, K., Bennett, D. S., & Carvalho, K. S. (2014). Attention deficit hyperactivity disorder and sleep disordered breathing in pediatric populations: A meta-analysis. *Sleep Medicine Reviews*, *18*(4), 349–356. https://doi.org/10.1016/j.smrv.2013.12.003.

Sleep Foundation. (2020, September 24). *Sleep strategies for children*. Sleep Foundation. Retrieved August 29, 2021, from https://www.sleepfoundation.org/children-and-sleep/sleep-strategies-kids.

Sullivan, C. E., Berthon-Jones, M., Issa, F. G., & Eves, L. (1981). Reversal of obstructive sleep apnoea by continuous positive airway pressure applied through the nares. *The Lancet*, *317*(8225), 862–865. https://doi.org/10.1016/s0140-6736(81)92140-1.

Taheri, S., Lin, L., Austin, D., Young, T., & Mignot, E. (2004). Short sleep duration is associated with reduced leptin, elevated ghrelin, and increased body mass index. *PLOS Medicine*, *1*(3). https://doi.org/10.1371/journal.pmed.0010062.

Tobias, L., & Won, C. (2016). Pro: Upper airway resistance syndrome represents a distinct entity from obstructive sleep apnea syndrome. *Journal of Dental Sleep Medicine*, *03*(01), 21–24. https://doi.org/10.15331/jdsm.5366.

UCAR. (2014). *Oxygen*. Oxygen | UCAR Center for Science Education. Retrieved August 29, 2021, from https://scied.ucar.edu/learning-zone/air-quality/oxygen.

Varga, M. D. (2012). Adderall Abuse on College Campuses: A Comprehensive Literature Review. *Journal of Evidence-Based Social Work*, *9*(3), 293–313. https://doi.org/10.1080/15433714.2010.525402.

Watson, N. F., Badr, M. S., Belenky, G., Bliwise, D. L., Buxton, O. M., Buysse, D., Dinges, D. F., Gangwisch, J., Grandner, M. A., Kushida, C., Malhotra, R. K., Martin, J. L., Patel, S. R., Quan, S. F., & Tasali, E. (2015). Recommended amount of sleep for a Healthy Adult: A joint consensus statement of the American Academy of sleep medicine and sleep Research Society. *Journal of Clinical Sleep Medicine*, *11*(06), 591–592. https://doi.org/10.5664/jcsm.4758.

Zulauf, C. A., Sprich, S. E., Safren, S. A., & Wilens, T. E. (2014). The complicated relationship between Attention Deficit/Hyperactivity disorder and substance use disorders. *Current Psychiatry Reports, 16*(3). https://doi.org/10.1007/s11920-013-0436-6.

CHAPTER SIX

feel and think

BRAINIAC-YAK-YAK

INTRODUCTION

This chapter is on *emotional*, *social*, and *cognitive health*, and you might wonder why I feel even remotely qualified to write on this. We are all armchair psychologists, and because my mom was the real deal, I do know the difference. I am not an expert in all-things-psychological, but I've seen a lot. So much of children's health decline stems from an inability to resourcefully respond to emotional curveballs. Stress is all around us—that's a given. And helping children learn how best to respond to stress, even the stress we create for them, is one of the Brave Parent's biggest challenges in life.

When it comes to emotional health, most parents in our culture seek common goals: to grow emotionally healthy children, each with the confidence to chart his or her own unique course, to establish and maintain positive relationships, to develop the ability to consistently make responsible decisions, and to dodge the bullets of addiction and/or mental illness.

Each of us, with our own baggage, is doing the best we can, but let's face it. These babes don't come out of the womb with their own

205

handbooks, and even if they did, our personal flaws would periodically throw us a wrench. Being a Brave Parent doesn't mean being righteous. Once we accept our own imperfections, we can lighten up on some of the cruel judgments we render on our children.

My best advice here: Keep your eye on the prize! Grown-up children who have become their best, most authentic selves are kind to themselves and others, refrain from the constant comparison to others (which is an insidious cultural norm), can navigate their conflicts peacefully, and have the courage to ask for help when they need it. For most of us, it's the toughest job we'll ever have.

In this section we will talk about loving and intentional parenting, character development, the challenges of socialization in a digital world, social responsibility, stress reactions, addiction, anxiety, and depression. Since the 1990s we've witnessed a growing list of stressors along with amplified stress reactions among tweens and teens.

As I write this, we are in the midst of a worldwide COVID pandemic that has added significant stress, fear, and anxiety to children and adults who are desperately trying to cope with a multitude of work-life-home changes. It's reported that anxiety among Americans has risen from 20% to 40% in a year—though consensus among my physician colleagues suggests that report is far too modest.

Even before the pandemic, the rates of anxiety and stress had been increasing substantially in children and adolescents. Between 2001 and 2004, a survey was used to screen for psychiatric conditions in more than 10,000 teens. Even by 2004, one teen in every four met the diagnostic criteria for an anxiety disorder.

Chronic anxiety often contributes to depression, stress, and various pain syndromes, and according to the American Psychological Association (APA), irritability, anger, and depression are often the most common symptoms of stress in teens.

I've personally suffered nine of my kids (my patients) lose their lives by succumbing to suicide or street drug addiction. This upward-trending tragedy is *real* among our youth, and it begs more *real* solutions. We need more feet-on-the-street efforts to help parents, teachers, and all health care professionals recognize early symptoms. We must also expand our current capacity to meet the mental health challenges of our younger children ... *before* there is an addiction or crisis.

These chapters are meant to empower you with Brave Parent concepts to raise authentic, happy, and confident children.

6.1 OUR FIRST JOB IS TO DEEPLY LOVE THEM

Parenting is a humbling sport. It feels like there is no end to the weighty decision-making we're called to do every day. A few years before I had my son, Hunter, I attended a lecture by M. Scott Peck, author of *The Road Less Traveled,* and I kept his reassuring words as my mantra: "You can make a lot of mistakes with children, and they will likely turn out just fine—as long as you *deeply, genuinely love* them. Conversely, you can do everything just as you should, following all the 'best' parenting rules, but without genuine love, they will be much more likely to fail in life." He further recommended *listening* to your child, as an act of love. When your kiddo feels heard and understood, no matter what decision you make, it will ultimately register as one conspiring for their best.

I had my own moments as a parent. I was *always* sure of my good intentions and my love for Hunter. I *frequently* felt pleased about our dialogues and my decisions. And I *sometimes* felt like I just really blew it! Can you relate to that? Now, as the parent of adult-Hunter, I see such kindness and decency in him, a reflection of my personal core values. But I also recognize the cultural messages with which I burdened him. If I had it to do again, I would try to de-emphasize what behaviors and activities would please *me,* shifting my focus even further toward helping Hunter develop his own innate strengths. His uniqueness. For example, I'm a helper and peacemaker, and he is exceedingly competitive. I regret trying to massage his competitive spirit in an attempt to make him more amiable.

"

We **need** more feet-on-the-street **efforts to help** parents, teachers, and all health care professionals recognize *early symptoms.*

We must also **expand** our current capacity to meet the **mental health** challenges of our younger children ... **before** there is an **addiction** or **crisis**.

"

I would spare many of the messages about what we (as a society) expect of boys versus girls and men versus women. Instead, I would intentionally focus on what it looks like to be a really good human: a good citizen of our family, our community, our natural environment, and our world, regardless of his gender.

6.2 HELPING YOUR CHILD DEVELOP CHARACTER

Kids thrive when they're given limits, daily structure, and clear expectations. They want to be held accountable to a structure, even when they complain about it. Consistently living within the reasonable boundaries you set forth teaches children how to be better citizens and how not to lie, cheat, or steal from one other. But none of this is news to you. As you talk to your children about these goals, always try to examine your own behavior. You can really help them build integrity and moral character if you are a parent who walks the talk—living your integrity and moral responsibility to others.

A close friend came to me for advice, shocked when her teenage children were caught repeatedly sneaking their friends into their country club, over the back fence. She was in a quandary about what the consequences should be. It was a hard conversation because I couldn't help but remember five years prior, when she decidedly underpaid for her kids' entrance to a major amusement park by asking them to lie about their age. Many of us have made these inadvertent mistakes, hoping to get a little advantage here or there—and in doing so we teach our children what's considered "acceptable" behavior. I encouraged her to have a transparent conversation about it, which she did.

It's never too late to fess up, to own your own shortcomings, and to agree to work on your own integrity, character, and principles right along with your children. Demonstrating humility and saying, "Look, we're all human. Let's work on this together," is a priceless opportunity.

> "Kids *thrive* when they're given **limits**, daily **structure**, and clear **expectations**. They want to be held *accountable* to a structure, **even when they complain about it.**"

Grit is another concept that deserves teaching and modeling. It's a combination of perseverance, effort, and passion for a particular long-term goal or end state.

Remember the old adage, "If at first you don't succeed, try ... try again!" It feels good to master something quickly, but it feels so much better to achieve something great through long-term commitment and striving to succeed. Ultimately, we don't want to tell our children we're proud of them because they got it right, but we're proud of them, and happy for them, because they never gave up. If you want to grow your grit skills, look at the book *Grit: The Power of Passion and Perseverance* by pioneering psychologist Angela Duckworth.

Kids also need to mend their own fences. Sometimes I think we fail to pull back as our children are developing their own social awareness. Responding to our current culture of stranger danger, we choose our kids' playmates, plan their playdates, set specific rules of engagement, drive them to and from their adult-organized sports, and even solve their social conflicts. Granted, it's all with the intention to spare them from harm and hurt feelings. But in overstepping, we take away their opportunity to learn social responsibility—to help them develop skills that become eminently important, even by their middle school years when they begin to choose their own friends. They need to have the space to know they can do it on their own.

I have been deeply impacted by Dr. Brené Brown, an emotions researcher who, in her famous TED Talk on vulnerability and shame, spoke these words about kids:

"They're hardwired for struggle when they get here ... Our job is not to say, 'Look at her, she's perfect!' ... Our job is to look, and say, 'You know what? You're imperfect and you're wired for struggle, but you are worthy of love and belonging!' That's our job! Show me a generation of kids raised like that, and we will end the problems I think we see today."

If you're not familiar with her work, you'll definitely want to read

The Gifts of Imperfect Parenting: Raising Children with Courage, Compassion, and Connection, among her other wonderful books.

Not unlike Brené Brown, my mom was a reputable relationship therapist with a passion for continuing her doctoral education. In our home there was no feeling left unexplored. As my brother, Jim, and I learned to speak, read, write, swim, and ride a bike, our mom also included lessons in emotional health. There was a focus on helping us sort out our feelings and developing a language to describe them. Don't get me wrong, this was *not* entirely cool. At times it felt like it was too much work, and other times, too much infringement. Analogous to hand-me-down clothing, however, most of it felt too big for us when we got it, but we eventually we grew into it. Today we are in our sixties, and these pieces are treasured relics, sewn into the very fabric of who Jim and I are as adults.

In that vein, our mom continually impressed upon us how critical it is for *each child* to grow up with *at least one adult* who really "sees" them and truly loves them ... *despite* their human shortcomings! When Jim and I were old enough to choose our closest circle of friends, and later when we each started dating, she reiterated this advice: Try to choose partners who were well-loved by at least one adult during their primary years. She believed (from her experience and the literature) that love-deprived children have a deep void, for which they will look to their partner to fulfill. She was convinced however, that for most of them, a deep sense of love and belonging would always elude them.

If I'm describing you, you have my compassion. Be kind to yourself, as it's not your fault. Remember that a good therapist can fast-forward your growth and development and help you find the self-love you seek. This will make you an even better parent.

" In that vein, our mom continually impressed upon us how **critical** it is for each child to grow up with at least *one adult* who really **"sees" them** and **truly loves them** ... despite their human shortcomings. **"**

Most of us don't learn the language of social and emotional health from our parents. For good or for bad, we learn mostly by modeling our adult caregivers' behaviors. If you are a parent who overdramatizes emotions, your child will likely learn to do the same. Conversely, if you are stoic and avoid showing your emotions, your child will likely learn to diminish or bury their feelings. This can lead to patterns of emotional suppression, denial, and blaming.

The good news in today's world is that social and emotional learning (SEL) *can* be taught. Even if you are not good at it, there are valuable resources to help you learn along with your child. We can collectively teach our children how to understand emotions, set and achieve positive goals, manage conflicts, and make wise personal decisions around socialization. That is indeed how we will diminish bullying, exclusion, anxiety, and depression in our culture. Dr. Marc Brackett, author of *Permission to Feel* and *Emotional Literacy in the Middle School*, is a huge proponent of this concept.

As a side note, you might want to keep the SEL dialogue going with school administrators also. I can only imagine how our world might look if we included this in core curricula everywhere. If you are courageous enough to propose social and emotional learning to your child's superintendent or school board, consider me your cheer-leader. But first, arm yourself with a good look at Brackett's work.

If you have school-age children, watch (or re-watch) the 2015 Pixar movie *Inside Out*. The movie takes place in the head of an eleven-year-old girl named Riley during a stressful time in her life. There are five emotions—joy, sadness, anger, fear, and disgust—that take on their own characters, and they help Riley explore and navigate her world. Some of the lessons here are the importance of recognizing different emotions and finding language for them, communicating our emotions and ideas to others, and realizing that we *all* grapple with an array of mixed emotions.

6.3 FOSTERING A HABIT OF INTEGRITY

I define integrity for children simply:

Say what you mean and do what you say.

Teaching kids the value of truth-telling and promise-keeping is a continual challenge in today's world, where little white lies are what we've come to consider "tactful" communication.

Growing kids with a good self-esteem is a big deal, and growing integrity is part of that. While we could hand over their self-esteem by showering them with positive affirmation, it just doesn't work. What *does* work is acknowledging them as they string together one good decision after another—and that includes telling their truth and keeping their word.

There's a non-profit organization to support Brave Parents in growing these critical habits, for themselves and their children. It's called *because I said I would.* The company's founder, Alex Sheen, is one of world's foremost experts on accountability and commitment. His story is compelling. Alex launched the effort as a tribute to his father, who he considered the best promise keeper he'd ever known.

Since his father's passing on September 4, 2012, *because I said I would* has distributed over thirteen million promise cards to 178 countries. (A promise card is a practical tool that really can help you and your kids learn how to keep commitments.) I encourage you to spend some time exploring their website, becauseisaidiwould.org.

6.4 SOME STUFF ABOUT "STUFF"

As sad as it is, we live in a world where material belongings have been equated with the measure of our worth. So, most of us have succumbed to societal pressures to buy our kids lots of cool stuff. Beautiful clothes, most desirable toys, designer labels, the best sports equipment, a bigger TV, the most recent cell phones, etc. In fact, we often use our multitude of gifts as expressions of love.

Here's an example. When I travel with my team members to

another state for a continuing education conference, they remain preoccupied with the need to find something "just right" to bring back for each child, as a souvenir of their trip. Trust me when I say, it seems to cloud the entire trip with a hint of frustration. Then upon our return, it's not unusual to see them scatter with a frenzy throughout the airport to settle for *something* to bring home. I have come to recognize that this obligatory gift is a way to say, "I'm sorry for being gone." As I write this, I'm not at all sure my team members realize these are guilt-driven gifts, but the ritual is not about to change any time soon. And by now, their kids have been programmed to expect them.

A different approach might be to explain to their children that the trip was for their own personal growth, professional learning, and reenergizing. In that light, a different way of gift-giving might be to buy a personal treasure only if they happened to see something "just right" for their child along their travels. In that special, unexpected way, it might serve as an I-thought-about-you-when-I-saw-this kind of gift.

I see this example as a metaphor for the bigger picture. Giving our kids all kinds of "stuff" has become an attempted substitute for our *time*. Let's face it, the busier we are juggling work life, household tasks, other relationships, and self-care, the less time we have for one-on-one parenting. The busier we are, the more not-enoughness guilt and shame we carry.

The problem is "stuff" is a lousy replacement for your time. And your kids realize this. While buying sprees might appease your guilt, they teach kids the exact opposite values you hold dear, such as kindness, communication, family, and fun.

Plus, a focus on having the right "stuff" teaches kids how to feel *entitled*. They develop expectations about what they'll be given. Later, when it's time to be off your payroll, they often sacrifice their financial responsibility for their perceived material "needs." Young adults buying stuff on credit, with high (and compounding) interest rates, begins another downward spiral of anxiety, guilt, and shame.

So, resist the urge. Try instead to funnel the time and money you might squander on shopping into experiences. Go home empty-handed and give your child simple face-to-face *white space*. Take a hike, look at the stars, plan an art project, play games, read books together, dance, sing, and tell stories. Let these be the special gifts you build your child's values around.

6.5 SOCIALIZATION IN TODAY'S WORLD

I hear adults complain that "kids today ... they just don't look you in the eye anymore." What's true is that social norms have changed. The eye-to-eye connection, a smile (real or fake), and a firm hand-shake has customarily been replaced by a quick glance up from an electronic handheld, a head nod, and a "Hey." At first blush, it appears that kids today are just tuned out, but don't be fooled. Our deep need for meaningful human connection is stitched into our DNA. We *all* long for it. So, it's not that tweens and teens are less social than past generations, it's more likely they're *virtually* connected to thirty-three other peers ... at the same time. And it's not going to change any time soon.

Cell phones are amazing! They're not really phones though, are they? They are full-fledged computers with access to anything and everything on the internet. Children are intrigued by new informa-tion, from the mundane to the ingeniously novel and, yes, to the seductively provocative. They (and we) crave our connections to "friends," but it's obviously a slippery slope. Just like adults, it doesn't take much for kids to literally get *addicted* to the ding of the technology feed. It can be video games, incessant text messages, Snapchat, Instagram, microblogging, music videos, livestreaming, chatting/meeting apps, or whatever else strikes their friend-group fancy. When you feel frustrated that your child is glued to their phone, remember that it's *your* generation who created this tech-nology—and *you* who purchased it and gave it to your child. That's a reality we live with.

If you haven't yet watched the Netflix movie *The Social Dilemma*, do it. In this documentary-style film you will see just how dangerous the impact of social networking has been. Millennial tech experts sound the alarm on their own constructions. Most memorable for me was the declaration that these parent-age social media creators now refuse to allow their own kids to partake! Their distress is a good reminder that, as a parent, you ultimately still hold the reins on your child's exposure ... as long as you're the one paying the bill.

Most of us will seek a compromise, trusting that with age-appropriate parental guidance, social networking technology won't wreck your child. You can work with teachers to help assure that handheld devices are not allowed during classroom learning. At home, perhaps you balance screen time with play time, encouraging other gratifying activities. Generate a list of possibilities with your child such as enjoying nature, face-to-face outdoor play, pickup games, crafts, puppet shows, music performances, and/or creative, fun events with neighborhood kids.

Don't allow your child's screen time to be private. There are countless traps that can derail them, such as dangerous stranger chat (and other privacy infringements), intense social pressure to be "liked," and the cruelty of blaming or bullying without intervention. In short, your child's device usage deserves your attention!

Take inventory of your kids' apps and take it upon yourself to research the best practices. Talk to them about potential consequences since you can see pitfalls that they cannot. Do your best *not* to succumb to your child's complaints about how much freedom their friends have and why they deserve more privacy.

6.6 FRIEND-TO-FRIEND CONNECTIONS

Consider the tremendous challenge of teaching children to seek out genuine caring relationships, where they become considerate friends who choose not to be destructive but keep a strong voice that speaks to their own selves, their own values.

The early years are training grounds for adolescence, where they will continually be challenged to stand their ground in the face of peer pressure. That takes courage. But even then, the cost of staying silent about wrongdoings among their friends can be brutal.

In the fall of eighth grade, I walked away from a small group of my "best girlfriends" who were smoking weed on the way to school each morning. In the spring of eighth grade, I walked away from my next group of "best girlfriends" because they formed a stealing club I didn't want to be part of. They were going to allow me to be their friend without being in the club as long as I stole at least one item so they could be assured I wouldn't tell on them. I did it. In the dressing room of Jacobson's junior department, I put on the cheapest T-shirt I could find underneath my sweatshirt and walked right out the door, back to the middle school. The events that followed, including sleepless nights, returning the shirt to the department store manager, dumping my friend-group, and confessing to my parents, were full of grueling and indelible lessons that kept me company for years. I had help. Each of my parents seemed proud of how I handled my missteps and wrapped their arms around me with such compassion.

I'm grateful I had the internal fortitude and external support to bring it forward. The biggest moral dilemma was whether to report my friends to the manager who asked me directly. I chose not to.

> **❝** Our children's **worst decisions** are often accompanied by *shame*.
> And the cost of **staying silent** is huge.
> Talking it through helps your child make their *act* shameful ... not their *person*. **❞**

Our children's worst decisions are often accompanied by shame. And the cost of staying silent is huge. Talking it through helps your child make their *act* shameful ... not their *person*.

If you want to be the kind of parent to whom your children will confess their struggles, my advice is to build experiences from a young age where you consistently tie the natural consequences to their actions—and *don't* impose unrelated punishment. For example, when your child breaks something of value as a result of aggressive haphazard play, help them figure out how to fix it or pay for the replacement. Don't ground them by taking away other privileges. Read more on this from Jim Fey's *Love and Logic* book series.

I also like teaching the message, "In our family, we don't keep *secrets* ... only delightful *surprises*." You'll come to know the value of that idea if your child ever happens to be bullied, abused, drawn into a dangerous collusion, or inappropriately touched by someone. You will want to know about it, rather than having them harbor a dangerous secret because someone outside your family swore them to secrecy.

6.7 DEPRESSION AND SOCIAL MEDIA

Today's children yearn for constant *virtual* connection. Unfortunately, the literature leaves no question that an increase in social media use is significantly associated with an increase in depression. What's going on here?

It is not surprising that children's views of themselves and the world are heavily influenced by their internal responses to their daily social media posts. It's nearly impossible for them not to compare their reality to what they see others posting. Comparison is the enemy of joy.

SCREEN TIME

66 Don't allow your child's **screen time** to be private. There are countless traps that can derail them, such as **dangerous** stranger chat (and other privacy infringements), intense social pressure to be "liked," and the cruelty of **blaming** or **bullying** without intervention. In short, your child's device usage deserves your *attention!* **99**

Bullying has trended upward in today's world also, including *cyberbullying* in the social media world. The National Centre Against Bullying defines bullying as "an ongoing and deliberate misuse of power in relationships through repeated verbal, physical, and/or other social behavior that intends to cause physical, social, and/or psychological harm. It can involve an individual or a group." Social bullying can create immediate harm and long-lasting scars for those involved, including bystanders.

Social media posting makes it easier to launch wounding remarks because we don't need to see the fear on someone's face or the pain in their eyes before we push "send." Labeling, judging, and blaming people in hit-and-run confrontations invites defensiveness, denial, and emotional pain.

Pay attention to changes in your child's mood, sleep patterns, appetite, and social withdrawal and encourage your child to open up about what's happening. Listen calmly without judgment or inter-ruption and encourage them to uncover the whole story.

6.8 SOCIAL RESPONSIBILITY

It's impossible to avoid your child's exposure to social media, so it's best to teach them about social responsibility. Let's focus on the values of integrity, respect for all people, kindness, and the practice of healing apology.

INTEGRITY: Doing the right thing for the sake of doing the right thing. Every time. Every one of us encounters difficulties in life, and some of them are a direct result of our mistakes. But it is exponen-tially easier to forgive yourself if, looking back, you feel you did the right thing in the moment. Help your child make a *habit* of doing the right thing. Keeping lines of communication open—so they report their triumphs *and* their misjudgments—is tough in families where the imposed penalties for mistakes are brutal. Living in a high-handed culture teaches children to lie. Better is to find ways to let children suffer the *natural consequences* of their actions, and you serve as their compassionate ally, helping them strategize how they will get through it. I've learned so much about positive discipline from Jim Fay, author of many books including *Love and Logic*. In raising Hunter, it often took some creativity to tie in natural consequences for his wrong choices, but it was so much more effective than imposing an unrelated punishment, including "grounding."

RESPECT FOR ALL PEOPLE: Our current culture seems to be in a serious deficit here, and we can remedy this if we work with children about how to appreciate differences and variety among humans. Help them recognize that each of us grows up in different surroundings, using distinctive communication language and styles, expressing varying degrees of conflict, practicing very different belief systems/spiritual influences, maintaining diverse types of traditional celebrations, with family members with dissimilar sexual orientations, and sometimes expressing strong political affiliations. We can all do our part to judge others a little bit less every day of our lives. In that vibe, continuing to model respectful social responsibility for your children is even more effective than talking about it.

KINDNESS: I recently saw my favorite T-shirt that reads, "Kind people are my kind of people!" Shortly before his death, at age ninety-four, I remember seeing an interview with Dr. Benjamin Spock, arguably the most influential child-rearing expert of multiple generations. When asked the question, "Dr. Spock, if you were to write your book over again today, what, if anything, would you change?" He looked thoughtfully and answered very clearly, "I would include a lot more *kindness*." If we are lucky enough to live to a wise age of ninety-four, I suspect we will each look back and wonder how we could have been more kind to more people. Remember the words of Robin Williams: "Everyone you meet is fighting a battle you know nothing about. Be kind, always!"

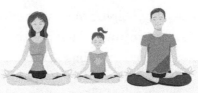

" To help soften your and your child's hearts, it helps to adopt an ongoing practice of **loving-kindness meditation,** or **metta**, as it is called in the Pali language. Through **visualization** and **meditation** phrases, metta teaches *how to love* all living beings **with wisdom** that has *no conditions*. It doesn't depend on whether one "deserves" it or not. It begins with **loving ourselves**, for unless we have a measure of this **unconditional love and acceptance** for ourselves, it is difficult to extend it to others. Then it expands to others who are special to us—parents, siblings, other family members, and friends—and ultimately, to *all living things*. "

Kindness can be instilled at a young age. We want our children to learn how to be kind to themselves first, their family members next, and *all* other living beings as well. That's often hard to do when siblings and parents seem like easy targets of our angst. From the time I was born my Gramma Kitty had this poem on her refrigerator that Jim and I were expected to memorize at a very young age:

> "We have a *smile* for
> the passing stranger,
> A kind *word* for
> the sometimes guest;
> But oft for our own, the bitter tone,
> Tho' we *love* our own the best!"

Those words stay with me to this day and now belong to my son, nephews, and nieces.

It's not too old-fashioned to teach your child the golden rule: *Do unto others as you would have them do unto you.* Look for real examples to dialogue about, asking them to reflect on how it might feel if that was done/said/posted about them.

To help soften your and your child's hearts, it helps to adopt an ongoing practice of loving-kindness meditation, or *metta*, as it is called in the Pali language. Through visualization and meditation phrases, metta teaches how to love all living beings with wisdom that has no conditions. It doesn't depend on whether one "deserves" it or not. It begins with loving ourselves, for unless we have a measure of this unconditional love and acceptance for ourselves, it is difficult to extend it to others. Then it expands to others who are special to us—parents, siblings, other family members, and friends —and ultimately, to all living things.

On a personal note, having a pet to care for is a good way to teach loving-kindness too. Dogs especially. Not only does having a dog in your home help strengthen your child's immune system (refer back to chapter 3 Digest), but in my opinion, they offer the best living example of unconditional love on the planet. No matter what mistakes we make, they love us back wholeheartedly! It is no wonder "dog" is "God" spelled backward.

> **66 Healing apologies** are thoughtful, genuine, and without defensiveness. *Remember* that the **best way to teach** this is to **exemplify it. 99**

LEARNING TO APOLOGIZE: I'm giving this its own space because I think the act of apologizing has become culturally muted. Our current society leans away from apologizing and accepting responsibility, toward blaming others and denial of responsibility. It's truly missing from politics and the media, also scant among social media posts and in business. So don't expect that your children will learn how to *own and apologize* anywhere but in their own home.

Why is it so important? Authentic apologies *heal*. They obviously go a long way to mend broken relationships because when we own our own part of the damage or disconnect, the other person feels understood. That alone is an act of loving-kindness. More importantly, authentic apologies between people often bring with it true *forgiveness*. Releasing the hurt, anger, and betrayal you felt toward someone else is really a gift we give ourselves.

I recently had an intimate dialogue with a longtime patient (and friend) Brenda. Her son Robbie was tragically killed in the eighth grade by a drunk driver. Now, after more than a decade, the man responsible for Robbie's death was released from prison, and Brenda was able to meet with him face-to-face. She wanted desperately to *forgive* him. She confessed to me the ugly thoughts she had toward him in the first years of her loss, but in her own journey toward healing she was able to see his tragic mistake as one she could ultimately forgive. It was no surprise that he was also needing to give her an authentic apology. With tears of joy, she said that this giving and receiving was perhaps one of truest gifts she'd ever bestowed upon herself.

So, I beg you—teach your child the power of a sincere apology. One that comes from the whole heart. We've all received halfhearted apologies that don't feel apologetic at all, and we can feel the difference. *Healing apologies* are thoughtful, genuine, and without defensiveness. Remember that the best way to teach this is to exemplify it. When you recognize *any* thought process or behavior that becomes important to your values and relationships, it's best to start with you, and invite others in. You might consider becoming accountability partners with your child (or entire immediate family) where you champion each other for extending an authentic apology and also grant permission to gently remind each other when an apology might be due.

6.9 THE REPTILIAN BRAIN AND THE THINKING BRAIN

Did you ever notice that during times of sudden threat, stress, or embarrassment, you just can't think straight enough to find the right words? That is called amygdala hijack—when your thinking brain is overruled by your ancient or reptilian brain. The amygdala, an almond-shaped part of the reptilian brain located at the base of the brainstem, drives our most basic needs. It continually scans the universe looking for answers to three protective functions:

1) Can I eat it? (Fulfilling hunger/thirst)
2) Will it eat me? (Ruling fear, anger, and aggression)
3) Can I have sex with it? (Ruling our need for procreation)

All of these functions are basic to our mere existence, so when the amygdala is triggered, it's totally charged! That's when we lose capacity to use the front of our brain—the prefrontal cortex—which is responsible for our ability to pay attention, not act on impulses, draw from past experiences, and have flexibility in our thoughts.

Why am I including this lesson in brain function? So you can recognize why your child might sometimes have difficulty accessing their best thinking. Adolescence is a time of enormously big social changes *and* hormonal changes. These are signs that your kiddo is forming an independent identity and learning to be an adult, but it also means they experience more frequent high-intensity positive and negative emotion. Meanwhile, sometimes they will temporarily lose the ability to use the front of their brain to consider potential consequences and make wise decisions.

It is up to you as a Brave Parent to recognize this and help them make sense of it—guide, secretly eyeroll, and wipe your brow. As they change, continue to remind them that, while you don't appreciate their behavior or decision, you love, love, LOVE them through it all.

The evidence is clear that our brains are growing and reshaping throughout our lives. It's called *neuroplasticity*. In response to learning or new experiences our brain has the ability to form and reorganize new circuitry, otherwise known as synaptic connections.

The saying that "neurons that fire together wire together" means that brain pathways, including what we believe and the way we behave, are functions of how pathways in the brain are formed and reinforced through repetition. For example, if you want to eat healthier, choose healthy foods and eat them for a month or two until your taste *preferences* reorganize to match your nourishing choices.

The best part of neuroplasticity is we can *relearn* anything by exercising new thought patterns. This is obviously useful following a traumatic brain injury or a supremely stressful event that results in post-traumatic stress syndrome. But it's also possible to help your child increase optimism, control anger, improve forgiveness, and experience more joy and fun in life. Let's take a look at stress first and then how best to respond.

6.10 STRESS REACTIONS IN CHILDREN

Stress in life is unavoidable, but too much stress is unhealthy. It's important to recognize stress reactions in your kiddos and equally important to teach coping skills along the way.

> **66** It's important to have a thorough **medical workup** to rule out the threat of **serious underlying illness** *before* attributing unusual symptoms to stress, **especially** when working with **infants** and **nonverbal children. 99**

Let me begin with a warning. It's important to have a thorough medical workup to rule out the threat of serious underlying illness before attributing unusual symptoms to stress, especially when working with infants and nonverbal children.

Stress is a ubiquitously used, big-bucket word that carries a thousand different connotations. Merriam-Webster's English Language Learners definition of stress is:

A state of mental tension and worry caused by problems in your life, work, etc.

The most commonly identified sources of stress in children are overscheduling, intrusion of technology into family time, two-working-parent families, the impact of divorce, abuse, acute or chronic pain, stranger or separation anxiety, school interruption (hello COVID pandemic), loss of control, loss of privacy, and loss of playtime.

These focus on stress from negative sources but be aware of stress from positive changes too. Like a new classroom, striving for peak performance on a sports team, efforts to maintain good grades, or being "liked" by a social group they desire.

Stress, whether positive or negative, induces ongoing physiologic effects of increased heart rate and blood pressure and elevated levels of stress hormones. There are three levels of stress to consider.

POSITIVE STRESS is within normal range *and* of limited duration. The first week of school is a good example for most children.

TOLERABLE STRESS is characterized by a high level of distress. An example is a serious illness (of your child or close family member) that is eased by the presence of loving, supportive family member relationships.

TOXIC STRESS is the highest level, marked by a prolonged duration, lack of supportive relationships, and sustained exposure to stress hormones. Toxic stress is labeled when it has clearly become associated with lifelong problems in behavior, learning, and mental and physical health.

Sometimes you will be aware of the source of your child's stress and sometimes not. They keep secrets out of fear of consequences, shame, embarrassment, fear of exposing others, or any number of other reasons. Even if a child perceives to be surrounded by empathic and nurturing family members, the very act of hiding the stressor(s) keeps these supportive family relationships just outside of reach.

It happened to me. My heart sank when Hunter, toward the end of his college years, admitted that he periodically felt bullied through elementary and middle school. I was shocked! I couldn't imagine why a smart, handsome, talented, and athletic guy like him would be bullied in the first place. (I realize this is probably a typical mom statement.) He was never one to complain so he kept it well hidden, which was not difficult. It was incredibly painful for me to hear just how he was tormented, and might I add, infinitely worse that I didn't learn of it until years after the fact! Just knowing he was alone in his suffering was enough to break my heart. I simply wasn't there to help him cope.

My point here is that your child's stress can be hidden, even when you think you have open communication.

Looking back, I feel grateful that he had a handful of good friends and family members who buoyed him, even when they didn't have a clue what was happening in the background. Fortunately for Hunter these episodes did not seem to result in toxic stress. That said, I believe that every act of human cruelty leaves a mark.

The bottom line is bullying is worth addressing as soon as you recognize it in your child or someone else's. Remember the old adage: If you see something, say something!

6.11 RAISING KIDS AS A SINGLE PARENT OR FROM TWO (OR MORE) HOUSEHOLDS

Sometimes by choice, and sometimes *not,* you might find yourself feeling alone in your efforts to parent ... or co-parent. I'm going to address co-parenting because for any child who goes back and forth between two households, alternating between very different modi operandi can create a level of stress all by itself. This includes situations of separation or divorce, death of a parent, a military parent deployed for periods of time, or being raised, in part, by grandparents.

It's often said that kids easily adapt to different rules in different homes. But when it comes to health training, it's much better to get on the very same Brave Parent page. Of course, that takes two parents who have good communication *and* a concerted effort to come together in a plan to raise healthy, happy kids. It's easier said than done! (I'm here to state the obvious: If harmonious communication was already in place, you might not be co-parenting from different households.) But never give up in your efforts.

I'm sure there's a ton of research on this subject, although I haven't done it. Mostly because *I lived it*, on both sides. I grew up amidst the consequences of divorce ... and so did my son. My parents divorced when I was three and a half. And setting a stereotypic example, I recapitulated the pattern, getting divorced when Hunter was virtually the same age. It was a painful chapter in all our lives.

Even today I want to say to twenty-seven-year-old Hunter, "I am so sorry, Honey. I know it wasn't always easy! But your dad and I did the best we could, trying not to have you pay the price for *our* personal mistakes."

And that's the point, isn't it? Not to have our children suffer an overt (or *covert*) war that marches on between two parents? I can tell you from firsthand experience, it felt like a blow to me, personally, whenever I would hear one of my parents insult the another. It's because I had such a sense of *belonging* to *both* of them that I took it so personally. Fortunately, that didn't happen often, but when it did, the derogatory comments were eked out in jest (which, by the way, didn't ease the sting).

In my dental office ... I regularly hear disparaging comments about who's at fault for this or that, pronounced *right* over the child.

Their beloved child is caught in a covert war, and I am always saddened by their pain.

Believe me, I'm not here to shame you if you decide to throw in the towel on a partnership. YOU deserve to be safe and happy. And so does your child.

> **66** While I **truly believe** *no child* goes **unscathed** by the *separation* of their **primary caregivers**, I also believe *no child* goes unscathed by **growing up** inside of a **torturous partnership**, of any kind. **99**

While I truly believe *no* child goes unscathed by the separation of their primary caregivers, I also believe *no* child goes unscathed by growing up inside of a torturous partnership, of any kind.

But I'm here to tell you, TIMES TWO, that it's very possible to come together as parents, despite some incredibly difficult challenges. Never give up on the idea of harmony. Here's the fantasy I create for parents who are in the throes of disharmony:

"Imagine waking up alone tomorrow, stranded on a deserted island, and discovering that the only other person on the island has nothing in common with you. You're doomed! And then you miraculously discover that they deeply love the very same person (a child, nonetheless) as much as you do! That commonality alone would be enough to bond you and sustain you. Your ongoing conversation would become rich with all the many successes—and also the challenges—that child was experiencing. It would be centered around how you wanted the absolute best for them."

Now come back to this world and bring your imagination with you. Why not try to keep your dialogue focused on the successes and challenges of your child ... whom you both love so dearly? And that includes putting together a mutually agreed upon plan for their health and happiness.

The same goes when, for your own reasons, you find yourself raising your child *singly*, within a village of devotees, rather than a two-parent household.

Whether through direct dialogue, phone, text, or email, keep re-centering your focus around your child's health and happiness. Let that take precedence over *all* other communications.

In that light, be sure to convey messages of celebration when something goes well, and humbly ask for help during challenging times. Remember, you will have a natural tendency to parent differently, as couples often do even within a stable marriage. But as you each deeply love your child, in your own ways, keep trying to let go of judgment and blame. In the absence of abuse (which demands your intervention), genuine love doesn't deserve our weighted judgment. Try assuming that the other is doing the best they can, under their own circumstances.

I am reminded of this quote by French essayist Joseph Joubert, "A part of kindness consists in loving people more than they deserve."

6.12 GETTING HELP FOR YOUR CHILD

In my integrative medicine training, I've been blown away by the abundance of scientific evidence surrounding mind-body techniques that can help reduce stress symptoms and related illness. These include breath work, progressive muscle relaxation, music therapy, guided imagery, loving-kindness meditation, yoga, and many other modalities.

I strongly advise that you choose health care providers who are qualified in a number of mind-body techniques as alternative (or adjunctive) therapy and who recognize these as respected options to antidepressant or antianxiety medications. I respect the role of psychotropic meds, but I find among my patients, they are often used as a first-line remedy. Drugs address symptoms but not the root cause(s). These less invasive techniques can help teach problem solving skills, reinforce health suggestions, and help them *choose* to respond to stress and anxiety in manageable ways.

Children can derive great benefit from learning to use mind-body techniques, and once learned, they can use them throughout their whole lives in a wide variety of settings. If you are a pediatric health practitioner, please approach their use with an open mind as to which technique might work best in any given situation. For example, some children are comfortable with imagery and storytelling, some will respond well to hypnosis (especially for pain management), and still others will triumph with the structure and visual cues of biofeedback.

If your child has a chronic health condition, practicing daily stress reduction is extremely helpful to reduce pain and stress. In fact, many of the best-studied target populations in pediatrics for mind-body interventions are among children with chronic conditions such as pain, arthritis, cancer, obesity, migraine or tension headache, recurrent abdominal pain, dysfunctional voiding, and inflammatory bowel disease. Mindfulness-Based Stress Reduction (MBSR) and Mindfulness-Based Cognitive Therapy (MBCT) are two of the most researched, non-pharmacologic modalities used successfully in children and adolescents dealing with health issues.

For pediatric practitioners knowledgeable about mind-body therapies, consider taking the lead in your community by educating your colleagues about these important techniques and advocating for school- and community-based programs to provide improved stress management options.

> **"**
>
> **Evidence** and **experience**
> indicate that all children have the
> potential to **benefit** from
> controlled **deep breathing**
> *Techniques.*
>
> Diaphragmatic (deep) breathing
> **stimulates** parasympathetic
> **relaxation**. That means it immediately
> **reduces heart rate** and **blood
> pressure**, helps the digestive system,
> and quells the **release** of
> *stress hormones.*
> **"**

Evidence and experience indicate that *all* children have the potential to benefit from controlled deep breathing techniques. Diaphragmatic (deep) breathing stimulates *parasympathetic* relaxation. That means it immediately reduces heart rate and blood pressure, helps the digestive system, and quells the release of stress hormones. Breathing has direct connections to emotional states and moods. Observe someone who is angry, afraid, or otherwise upset, and you will see a person breathing rapidly, shallowly, noisily, and irregularly. Conversely, you cannot be upset if your breathing is slow, deep, quiet, and regular! Just think about that. While we can't always emotionally re-center ourselves by an act of will, we can decide to make our breathing slow, deep, quiet, and regular. The rest will follow.

The best part about learning how to use breathing techniques for stress reduction is that children *always* have their breath. (By the way, so do we!) And it almost always works.

An easy technique to teach is four-count breathing. As you breathe in, count slowly up from *one* to *four*, fully filling your lungs. As you breathe out, count slowly back from *four* to *one*, fully emptying your lungs. Thus, as you inhale you say quietly to yourself, "One ... two ... three ... four," and as you exhale you say, "Four ... three ... two ... one." Repeat this several times.

6.13 SUSPECTED ABUSE AND POST-TRAUMATIC STRESS REACTIONS

Behavior changes or regressive behavior in children of any age may be a presenting sign of serious issues such as child abuse or post-traumatic stress disorder (PTSD). If you suspect a history of abuse or that your child has witnessed a traumatic event, it's important to schedule a consultation with a mental health specialist ASAP! Your child deserves a Brave Parent to advocate for them, procuring their safety and getting them help with the recovery process.

6.14 A CULTURE OF ADDICTION

Show me an adult without an addiction of some sort, and I'll show you a unicorn. I have learned how to caringly hack into people's lives, and I hear their stories of struggle with dependency. The word addict was derived from the Latin word *addictus* which means to devote, sacrifice, sell out, or enslave. For us, it's about craving something intensely, loss of control over its use, and/or continued involvement with it despite adverse consequences in one's life.

Addiction begins as a seductive pleasure and often ends in

tragedy. Thanks to my good friend, Dr. Robert Lustig, pediatric neuroendocrinologist and author of *Fat Chance, The Hacking of the American Mind,* and *Metabolical* (ALL worth the read!), I have developed a reasonable understanding of the addiction's downward spiral.

The feeling of pleasure is stimulated by a spurt of dopamine, a neurochemical transmitter in the part of the brain called the nucleus acumens—the brain's pleasure center.

Lustig helps us to differentiate happiness from pleasure. *Happiness* is regulated by a different neurochemical transmitter, *serotonin.* Our culture thrives on pleasure over happiness all day long. We crave the dopamine thrust and we go for it, hit by hit, through our behaviors, natural rewards such as food or sex, or psychostimulant substances we consume.

Dopamine regulates our emotional and motivation behavior. Psychostimulants, drugs of abuse, and natural rewards all can cause the reward-satisfaction system to go haywire. The pleasure associated with an addictive drug or a pleasurable behavior dwindles, and yet the memory of the desired effect and craving to recreate it persists.

Between sugar, caffeine, the ping of a cell phone, social media threads, electronic gaming, gambling, alcohol, tobacco, snacking, weed, porn, prescription mood-altering drugs, and opioids, it seems everybody's got some addiction—little or big. Ninety-three percent of adults refuse to wake up in the morning without caffeine and/or sugar. While sugar may seem the most innocuous on this list, I assure you, it's killing us. We're absolutely out of control with sugar, consuming an average of twenty-two teaspoons per person each day! That's fifty-seven pounds a year! To our detriment, sugar addiction wreaks havoc with weight stability, metabolic health, cardiovascular health, dental health, and the list goes on.

You're not surprised to hear that sugar is an addictive substance, are you? Turns out, it lights up the brain just like cocaine and has us craving more of it for less effect. Tragically, the food industry has been complicit with ratcheting upward our "bliss point." Yes, that is their word for hyper-palatability. It's defined as the amount of sugar, salt, and fat that peaks the pleasure center of the brain, stimulating the dopamine hit that causes us to crave more.

With drug addiction, it results in compulsive drug-seeking and drug-taking behaviors that continues despite even the most terribly destructive consequences. Mind-altering drugs can release two to ten times more dopamine than natural rewards do, and they do it more quickly and more reliably. The brain responds by producing less dopamine and eliminating some dopamine receptors. This is called *downregulation*, and it means you have to provide more of the stimulus to obtain the same dopamine "high." It also a creates an effect known as *tolerance*.

Every one of us wants desperately to avoid drug addiction for our children. I wish this book included a magic wand for that. It's helpful to educate your children to recognize signs of dependency in themselves and others, talk about it openly, and continually address any of your own drug addictions (prescription or recreational) with humility and grace.

The top six drugs causing addiction in the US are, in order, tobacco (nicotine), alcohol, marijuana, opioid pain killers, cocaine, and heroin.

If there are a few pieces of advice I can offer you from my observations of thousands of parents and kids, they are:

First, identify and address your own addictions so your child doesn't have to live with it as a model. This includes your dependency on alcohol and marijuana, tobacco, high doses of caffeine, sleeping pills, and pain killers.

Second, don't give your kids sleeping pills or pain killers! This sounds so obvious, doesn't it? But I commonly hear that parents are feeding their kids melatonin or Benadryl to wind down at night, after hyping up on sugar, caffeine, and/or prescription stimulants (for ADHD) during the day. Teaching kids to rely on chemical substances for waking and sleeping is a setup for future addiction.

You're not surprised to hear that **sugar** is an **addictive** substance, are you? Turns out, it lights up the brain just like **cocaine** and has us *craving* more of it for less effect. Tragically, the food industry has been complicit with ratcheting upward our **"bliss point."** Yes, that is their word for **hyper-palatability.** It's defined as the amount of sugar, salt, and fat that peaks the pleasure center of the brain, *stimulating* the **dopamine** hit that causes us to *crave more.*

Next, avoid pain medications (even acetaminophen and ibuprofen) for minor muscle aches and pains. Remember that pain is a natural biological feedback mechanism, signaling that something is injured or healing. Save pharmaceuticals for real pain. I'm not suggesting you don't use them to control a spiking fever or major pain, but again, don't teach children to over-rely on these for the little stuff.

And while we're on pain killers, don't let health professionals prescribe opioids for your kiddo unless the circumstances are dire. Remember that the first rush of an opioid for anyone is almost always powerfully pleasurable. This can create a neurochemical attraction they will chase later in life.

The first taste of an opioid "high" is often when kids get their wisdom teeth out. Just say "no thanks" to the follow-up prescription. I like to remind parents that ibuprofen is considered the best remedy for dental pain, and if that's not enough, alternating over-the-counter doses of acetaminophen *and* ibuprofen should temper it. I may seem overly anxious about this, but that's because I've watched dozens of my kids (patients) slip into opioid addiction the last fifteen years. The way I see it, if your teenager has to lie on the couch sober and be slightly uncomfortable for a bit, that's okay—after all, they just had teeth removed.

Finally, I loathe the recent trend of posting funny videos of your child "high" from the oral surgeon's IV sedation. (Parents, the unbrave kind, seem to participate in this all the time these days). Aggrandizing the experience as fun and pleasurable is absolutely the wrong message for kids *and* adults!

I would be remiss to end this section without addressing vaping —it has rather suddenly become all the rage in middle school and high school. Many drugs can be consumed through vaping and at the top of the list is nicotine, perhaps the most insidiously addictive molecule on the planet. According to a 2020 National Youth Tobacco Survey, 3.6 million US school-age kids use E-cigs—including one in five high schoolers. This growing epidemic should be shut down by illegalizing E-cigs, but if there's anything we know all too well, it's that the power of the tobacco industry is powerful. I urge you to look at TobaccoFreeKids.org and consider joining the fight. Meanwhile, please have a serious discussion with your kiddo about the sneaky nature of nicotine's ability to enchain them. What starts out seeming "cool" can quickly become a terrible burden.

6.15 ANXIETY

Anxiety is a normal emotion and one we all rely on for survival. It helps us prepare for challenges and avoid potentially threatening or dangerous situations. But it's also one of the most contagious emotions we experience. One flare can ignite a bonfire among a group. I notice that anxious children often get cues from an anxious parent. I see this emotional transference frequently in my office. If a child is highly anxious in the dental chair, nine times out of ten, they are accompanied by a parent with high dental anxiety.

If you suffer from anxiety, keep finding ways to improve your own anxiety. It will be a gift to your family.

Anxiety disorders are the most common mental illness in the US, affecting forty million adults every year. That's almost one in five of us. Sadly, the stats are even worse for teens. According to the NIH, nearly one in three of all adolescents (ages thirteen to eighteen) will experience an anxiety disorder. These data combined with the rate of hospital admissions for suicidal teens (also doubled over the past decade) leave me a little freaked out.

The staggering upward trend of my kiddos, toddlers to teens, who suffer from anxiety disorders might be the most marked heartbreaking trend I've witnessed in my career. Countless scholarly articles indicate a continual rise in prevalence of both anxiety and depressive disorders in adolescents over the last three decades. Then, just like that, they doubled during the COVID-19 pandemic. These trends cut across all demographics, in *all* industrialized countries.

66 The **staggering upward trend** of my kiddos, toddlers to teens, who *suffer* from **anxiety disorders** might be the most marked heartbreaking trend I've witnessed in my career.

Countless scholarly articles indicate a *continual rise* in the prevalence of both **anxiety** and **depressive** disorders **in adolescents** over the last three decades. Then, just like that, they **doubled** during the **COVID-19 pandemic.** 99

Anxiety disorders develop from a complex set of risk factors, including genetics, brain chemistry, personality, and life events. As with any chronic condition/illness, it is much better to catch them early.

When normal anxiety begins to keep children from experiencing the everyday joys in their lives, it is considered a disorder. Unfortunately, as a parent, it is often difficult to recognize anxiety disorders before they become catastrophic. Even when we take our glasses off to catch a glimpse, we tend to rationalize unusual behavior, put our blinders back on, and ignore what's right smack dab in front of us.

Some of the more common symptoms include concentration problems (similar to ADHD), sleep disturbance, waking with bad dreams, changes in appetite, frequent fidgeting, becoming tense or irritable, expressing constant worry, or having uncontrolled outbursts. You might also see unexplainable physical symptoms such as stomachaches, headaches, shortness of breath, chest pain, gagging, or vomiting. If you notice these, ask your child's physician or nurse practitioner to steer you in the right direction. If you're catching it early, medication should not be the first-line treatment.

I am entirely alarmed by the number of psychotropic medications prescribed for children. Many of my kiddos have been prescribed stimulants for ADHD when it may well be a sleep/breathing disorder or an anxiety disorder, *not* an attention deficit disorder at all. Some kids can't pay attention because they are too tired or worried, and if sleep deprivation is a problem, imagine how dosing a child with a stimulant twice a day might double their trouble. (Learn more on this by returning to the chapters on Breathe and Sleep.)

Antidepressants (SSRIs) are also frequently prescribed as first-line therapy for pediatric anxiety disorders, and now that marijuana is considered a viable treatment for anxiety, I see many parents who view weed as an acceptable treatment choice for their teens and young adults. There is reliable evidence that a young person's brain continues to develop into their early twenties, and using cannabis can have a permanently negative effect on brain development. And if you're using weed or alcohol to quell your own anxiety, just know that your child is learning how to rely on a drug instead of less invasive, more effective coping mechanisms.

By now you know that I'm not a big fan of our quick-to-medicate Western approach to most conditions. Meds usually quell the *symptoms* instead of helping at the *root cause* level. Fixing problems at the root cause level is usually less invasive and an all-around better solution.

I say that as if it were easy to do. It's not! But over the years I've noticed that medicating children for anxiety, without addressing their issues from a functional, behavioral, and psychological perspective can become a slippery slope to depression, dependency, and life-threatening addiction.

6.16 DEPRESSION

Sadness and grief are normal human emotions as well. We each have those feelings from time to time, especially in response to a significant disappointment, but normally they fade away within a few days, and we find ourselves experiencing emotions of happiness, pleasure, and even joy once again.

Major depression or *major depressive disorder* is something more serious. It's a diagnosable mood disorder that can bring about ongoing symptoms such as overwhelming sadness, low energy, loss of appetite, and a lack of interest in things that used to bring pleasure. If left unrecognized and/or untreated, depression can lead to serious health complications, including putting your child's life at risk.

How rapidly is major depressive disorder trending upward? Depression among kids ages fourteen to seventeen years old increased more than 60% between 2009 and 2017. This catastrophic rise is linked to a number of changing cultural factors, including increased time participating in social media.

66 It is criticial to recognize the signs of

childhood depression

and when you see them, **keep your blinders off!** It's scary for sure because we have a **built-in bias**—we want our kids to be healthy.

Depression is often **undiagnosed and untreated** because symptoms are passed off as normal **emotional and psychological** changes. **99**

Suicide is the second leading cause of death among American children thirteen to nineteen years old and tenth leading cause of death among all Americans. According to the CDC, 8.9% of high school students surveyed have *attempted* suicide and 18.8% of high school students *seriously considered* suicide.

It is critical to recognize the signs of childhood depression and when you see them, keep your blinders off! It's scary for sure because we have a built-in bias—we want our kids to be healthy. Depression is often undiagnosed and untreated because symptoms are passed off as normal emotional and psychological changes.

The primary symptoms revolve around prolonged sadness (lasting two weeks or more), feelings of hopelessness, bouts of unusual irritability, and mood changes. Acknowledge what you're seeing, but do it with compassion and without a hint of character judgment. If your child is met with constant criticism of their behavior change, they are more likely to mask their symptoms. Instead, stay curious about their feelings and model open communication by sharing your feelings too.

Growing up with a mom who was a relationship psychologist, I remember her giving me a list of emotions and talking through what each of them meant. It's an unusual vocabulary list for most kids, and at the time, I didn't understand why I needed that exercise. Looking back, I'm grateful. It was nice to be able to express the difference between emotions like sad, angry, hurt, offended, afraid, or jealous. I was also repeatedly encouraged (and praised) for expressing my own authentic voice in intimate relationships and for standing up for myself whenever I felt my character or integrity was being compromised. Maybe these exercises can be a way for you to help your child too. You might enjoy clinical psychologist Harriett Learner's book *The Dance of Connection: How to Talk to Someone When You're Mad, Hurt, Scared, Frustrated, Insulted, Betrayed, or Desperate.*

If you suspect major depression, pay particularly close attention to any expressed desires (verbal or visual) of self-harm. Research shows suicidal thoughts and behaviors are the greatest predictors of suicide.

Fortunately, there are several effective treatments for major depressive disorders, such as psychotherapy, mind-body therapies (as discussed above), diet alteration, regular physical activity, and antidepressant medications. Child psychologists and psychiatrists are in high demand, but be persistent. As the bravest of Brave Parents, rely on your child's primary care provider to help make a strong referral while you stand tall as their champion. Don't give up until they find a good fit with a well-trained health professional.

6.17 COGNITIVE LEARNING IN TODAY'S WORLD

I'm 100% dedicated to the practice of lifelong learning, and I try to inspire that concept in my kids (patients). In fact, when my high school and college kids ask my opinion about what they should do for a job, I like to answer, "What do you think you'd like to keep learning about?"

That's my best advice, given in a world where only 20% have passion for their work. Wouldn't you like your child to be one of them? To do so we need to make learning a daily craving.

One unique thumbprint of my *total health dental practice* is the way we foster health literacy for children. We treat them to a hands-on, health-related science experience at every preventive visit. The Hands-On Learning Lab™ concepts are challenging, but in our experience, *all* kids are good learners—and they *all* seem to enjoy it.

But when I ask these *same kids*, "How's school going?" I find the majority have grown to dislike the classroom by about the fourth grade ... and forevermore. Even my college kids (who seem enlivened by the social experience of student life) become almost disconnected from the learning itself. In short, most schoolchildren in today's world are just trying to slug through it, chasing a decent grade and hoping for as little work (in other words, as little *learning*) as possible.

When and *why* do kids turn the corner from enjoying learning to barely tolerating it?

Through a look at contemporary literature in cognitive and educational sciences, the problem has become apparent to me. People have been going about learning in wrong ways. And, as a result, kids just lose interest.

The challenge for you, as a Brave Parent, remains: What can you do to engage your child in learning so they grow up to be self-directed and even inspired? To make a long answer short ... We need to *make it harder, create spaced repetition,* and *make it "interleaved."* Don't worry, I will explain.

Before I do, let me express my deep respect for all schoolteachers everywhere. I'm oh so grateful for those passionate educators who (mostly) rocked the paradigm shift to virtual learning during the COVID pandemic. Many of them were educating your children while they were at home parenting their own. And most have transitioned back to in-person learning with grace. My intention is not to rifle them with these concepts, but to help us all take a new perspective on an inherent dilemma: the lack of engagement in the learning itself.

Cognitive science is an interdisciplinary study of the mind and intelligence, blending such factions as neuroscience, linguistics, psychology, anthropology, and philosophy. Scientists' recent conclusions about optimal learning help us to understand how children (and adults) learn better, remember longer, and become more self-directed. And what's really cool is we now recognize that the very elements that shape our cognitive abilities lie within our own control.

6.18 LEARNING THAT LASTS IS EFFORTFUL

The first important concept to consider is that making learning simple doesn't help it to stick. Think about your experience. Recall the many memorization tools you ever created that helped you regurgitate factual information for a quiz or a test. As you already know, they all worked ... for the test. Unfortunately, that kind of learning is here today and gone tomorrow. The most long-lasting learning is *difficult,* not easy.

As a Brave Parent you will want to help stimulate *desirable challenges*, meaning inherent difficulties that help engage your child's brain. Encourage your kiddo to *ponder the problem* before they formulate possible strategies and solutions. That way you're priming their mind for learning.

Difficult doesn't mean it can't be FUN at the same time. Keep the dialogue lively and entertain their most creative, zany ideas.

By the way, this concept is true for us too. Think of the many times you really grappled with how to solve a problem *before* you discovered the solution. Chances are you learned the solution by heart once it came to you. Take this book for example. I'm guessing your most memorable "ah-ha" moments are from answers to the quandaries you've been thinking about long before you turned the first page.

> **66** What can you do to **engage** your child in **learning** so they grow up to be **self-directed** and even *inspired*? To make a long answer short ... **We need to make it harder,** create spaced *repetition* and make it "**interleaved.**" **99**

So, from now on, whenever your child asks you for the answer to an unknown fact or a problem, take a minute or two to help them restate the quandary (or question) and explore their own imagined solutions (or answers). In that way, their brain becomes hungry for learning.

After engaging with your child about the nature of the problem, if you don't know the answer, consider it an opportunity to do some research *together*. It's much better to become a learn-it-all than a know-it-all! Do your best to model the behavior of a curious, continual learner, rather than trying to be seen as the resident expert on everything.

While your kiddo is wrestling with effortful learning, reassure them that, if it feels like it takes too much brain power, there's a pretty good chance you're onto some big learning ... and an even better chance you'll never forget it.

Not so incidentally, this concept really elevates the advantages of intellectual failures and setbacks—they are the scaffold from which to build a new strategy. Once your child's brain is frustrated and hungry for the solution, they will likely be open to a *new* strategy, and ultimately the learning will be much more deep-rooted.

> **66** While your kiddo is wrestling with **effortful learning**, reassure them that, if it feels like it takes too much *brain power*, there's a pretty good chance you're onto some big learning ... and an even better chance **you'll never forget it. 99**

6.19 PLEASE REPEAT THAT

Next is the concept of *repetitive retrieval*. My high school math teacher Mr. Steidel was a scholar and a philosopher. His favorite saying (in his Southern drawl) was, "Repetition is the mother of learnin'." It's no wonder that he repeated that almost daily, as he periodically re-reviewed the same mathematic principles with different variables. We learned them well and I think my entire class aced the AP Calc exam (circa 1978).

He got it right! Today the science supports Mr. Steidel. Turns out, *repetitive retrieval* of learned information helps cement the brain's circuitry. In other words, periodic repetition interferes with the act of forgetting.

That's opposite our cultural norm, which leans toward *massed learning*, a single, lengthy session of learning in preparation for a test and then a mind dump. We call this "cramming." *Yes*, cramming can procure a good test score, especially if you've had a good night's sleep instead of pulling an all-nighter. And *yes*, you can string these good scores together to earn a high grade in the class. But *no*, that doesn't mean you will retain your new knowledge over time.

Retention is even more beneficial if you study for shorter periods and repeat the lesson periodically over time. That's called *spaced* repetition. So, I'll say it again, for Mr. Steidel: "Repetition is the mother of learning."

To help your kids learn *everyday life lessons*, make spaced repetition your routine. And space out the retrieval practice. Try starting with daily repetition, for a couple days, then again in a week, then on to every few weeks, and eventually once a month. If your kids give you an I-already-know-this eyeroll, challenge them to teach it to someone else.

To help your kids with *classroom concepts*, try working with them to make flashcards or little quizzes covering key ideas, and put them away after a couple days. Then bring them back out weekly to interrupt their forgetting.

6.20 MIX IT UP

Another habit that helps kids cement their learning is called *inter-leaved practice*—when the brain is taxed to learn two (or more) *related* concepts or skills at the same time. The idea is to alternate between two or three related concepts, learning them in smaller chunks rather than studying them comprehensively, one at a time, in sequential order.

Examples of interleaved practice are studying a handful of grammatical rules (or a grouping of different math problems) by alternating between them.

With your kids, resist the urge to keep them solely focused on one effort to completion. Encourage them to practice multiple concepts each day by incorporating a mix of similar topics and by switching back and forth between them.

While you're getting the hang of this, consider applying these practices of spaced repetition and interleaved learning to the many Brave Parent lifestyle changes you might be making, for the sake of your child's health and happiness. In other words, don't be afraid to tackle a handful of significant changes at a time. You can teach them *why* you are implementing specific changes, *while* you overhaul your lifestyle.

If you want a deeper dive into these learning concepts, start by reading the book *Make it Stick* by Peter C. Brown and Henry Roediger III.

CONCLUSION

We all agree that social, emotional, and cognitive health are critically important in raising happy, healthy children. As parents, we walk a fine line between allowing independent decision-making and over-steering their journey. Remember, we're aiming for "roots and wings." We want our kids to be grounded in good character with the confidence to travel an uncharted path that is unique to only them. I love the painted sign by our door that reads "Go out for adventure, come home for love."

That said, your role as the brave, crusading, warrior parent means never taking your eye off the ball in areas of social, emotional, and cognitive health, even when your adolescent child is finding their independence. If you recognize an adverse change in your child's emotional or mental health, don't sweep it under the rug. You don't need to have all the answers. Seek professional help and collaborate with them for strategies that will make a difference. Remember, it takes a village to raise a healthy, happy child.

CHAPTER 6 REFERENCES

Adam, A. (2021). *Amygdala hijack: Symptoms, causes, and prevention.* Medical News Today. Retrieved October 20, 2021, from https://www. medicalnewstoday.com/articles/amygdala-hijack#summary.

APA. (2008). *APA Public Opinion Poll – Annual Meeting 2018.* APA Public Opinion Poll – annual meeting 2018. Retrieved October 15, 2021, from https://www.psychiatry.org/newsroom/apa-public-opinion-poll-annual-meeting-2018.

APA. (2020). *Stress in America™ 2020: A National Mental Health Crisis.* American Psychological Association. Retrieved October 15, 2021, from https://www.apa.org/news/press/releases/stress/2020/report-october.

Brackett, M. A. (2019). *Permission to feel: Unlocking the power of emotions to help our kids, ourselves, and our society thrive.* Celadon Books.

Brown, B. (2013). *The Gifts of Imperfect Parenting: Raising Children with Courage, Compassion, and Connection.* Sounds True, Incorporated.

Brown, P. C. (2018). *Make it stick: The science of successful learning.* Belknap Harvard.

Duckworth, A. (2016). *Grit: The power of passion and perseverance.* Scribner.

Feeney, K. E., & Kampman, K. M. (2016). Adverse effects of marijuana use. *The Linacre Quarterly, 83*(2), 174–178. https://doi.org/10.1080/00243639.2016.1175707.

Hathaway, W. R. (2021, June 11). *Neuroanatomy, prefrontal cortex.* StatPearls [Internet]. Retrieved October 16, 2021, from https://www.ncbi.nlm.nih.gov/books/NBK499919/.

Heid, M. (2019, March 14). *Depression and suicide rates are rising sharply in Young Americans, new report says.* Time. Retrieved November 2, 2021, from https://time.com/5550803/depression-suicide-rates-youth/.

Ivey-Stephenson, A., Demissie, Z., Crosby, A., Stone, D., Gaylor,

E., Wilkins, N., Lowry, R., & Brown, M. (2020). *Suicidal ideation and behaviors among high school students* ... Suicidal Ideation and Behaviors Among High School Students — Youth Risk Behavior Survey, United States, 2019. Retrieved October 27, 2021, from https://www.cdc.gov/mmwr/volumes/69/su/pdfs/su6901a6-H.pdf.

Juergens, J. (2021, October 27). *10 most common addictions.* Addiction Center. Retrieved November 1, 2021, from https://www.addictioncenter.com/addiction/10-most-common-addictions/.

Kessler, R. C., Berglund, P., Chiu, W. T., Demler, O., Heeringa, S., Hiripi, E., Jin, R., Pennell, B.-E., Walters, E. E., Zaslavsky, A., & Zheng, H. (2004). The US National Comorbidity Survey Replication (NCS-R): Design and field procedures. *International Journal of Methods in Psychiatric Research, 13*(2), 69–92. https://doi.org/10.1002/mpr.167.

Lerner, H. G. (2002). *The dance of connection: How to talk to someone when you're mad, hurt, scared, frustrated, insulted, betrayed, or desperate.* HarperCollins.

Lustig, R. H. (2017). *The hacking of the American mind: Inside the sugar-coated plot to confuse pleasure with happiness.* Avery.

Lustig, R. H. (2017). *The hacking of the American mind: The science behind the corporate takeover of our bodies and brains.* Avery, an imprint of Penguin Random House.

Marchand, W. R. (2012). Mindfulness-based stress reduction, mindfulness-based cognitive therapy, and zen meditation for depression, anxiety, pain, and psychological distress. *Journal of Psychiatric Practice, 18*(4), 233–252. https://doi.org/10.1097/01.pra.0000416014.53215.86.

Merikangas, K. R., He, J.-ping, Burstein, M., Swanson, S. A., Avenevoli, S., Cui, L., Benjet, C., Georgiades, K., & Swendsen, J. (2010). Lifetime prevalence of mental disorders in U.S. adolescents: Results from the National Comorbidity Survey Replication–Adolescent Supplement (NCS-A). *Journal of the American Academy of Child & Adolescent Psychiatry, 49*(10), 980–989. https://doi.org/10.1016/j.jaac.2010.05.017.

Peck, S. (2003). *The road less traveled.* Touchstone.

Stamm, K., Lin, L., & Christidis, P. (2018, March). *Mental disorders most frequently treated by psychologists*. Monitor on Psychology. Retrieved November 2, 2021, from https://www.apa.org/monitor/2018/03/datapoint.

Twenge, J. M., Cooper, A. B., Joiner, T. E., Duffy, M. E., & Binau, S. G. (2019). Age, period, and cohort trends in mood disorder indicators and suicide-related outcomes in a Nationally Representative Dataset, 2005–2017. *Journal of Abnormal Psychology, 128*(3), 185–199. https://doi.org/10.1037/abn0000410.

Weir, K. (2015, November). *Marijuana and the developing brain*. Monitor on Psychology. Retrieved November 10, 2021, from https://www.apa.org/monitor/2015/11/marijuana-brain.

CHAPTER SEVEN

chew and smile

ORAL HEALTH WISE ... THE MOUTH IS A TATTLETALE

INTRODUCTION

In my thirty-six years as a curious dentist, I have come to understand that a healthy mouth is indicative of a healthy body, and vice versa.

That means that oral disease negatively impacts our other organs. There are now fifty-seven systemic ailments associated with periodontal (gum) disease alone, including preterm, low birth weight babies and stillbirth, not to mention heart disease, dementia, depression, and pneumonia.

And the other way around, our bodies' systemic illnesses exhibit recognizable signs and symptoms in the mouth! For example, the very first signs of diabetes show up as bleeding gums, dry mouth, oral fungal infections (thrush), or even a change in the way you taste your food.

As a health educator, I travel around the country speaking to dental (and other) health professionals to help them clearly uncover the mouth's telltale signs of these systemic disorders and diseases.

For once they see them, they can't *un-see* them. If you want to learn more check out my first book, *BlabberMouth: 77 Secrets Only Your Mouth Can Tell You to Live a Healthier, Happier, Sexier Life,* and also *The Shift: The Dramatic Movement Toward Health Centered Dentistry* by Dr. DeWitt Wilkerson.

I will uncover some those mouth-body connections for you in the following pages, but first let me start by talking about TEETH!

Your kiddos' teeth are given to them in two sets. The practice set (spanning from six months old till about twelve years old), and the permanent set (spanning from six years old till their personal forever). That's right, their *permanent* teeth are supposed to be their chewers for a lifetime.

Now for a lesson in tooth anatomy. Imagine your tooth is analogous to an old-fashioned yellow pencil. The thin outer layer, *enamel,* is hard and protective, like the pencil's glossy yellow paint. The thick inner layer, *dentin,* is seven times softer than enamel—picture the wood core of the pencil. Finally, the inner *pulp* chamber. Just like the pencil lead, it occupies the central compartment of the tooth, and it contains the nerves and blood vessels that nourish the tooth.

There are many aspects of teeth that have perplexed me, and for many years, this was one of them. Tooth enamel is unlike any other part of our body's *ectoderm* (the body's outer covering that includes skin, hair, nails, and cornea of the eye). Enamel doesn't repair itself following injury or disease! That means, if you get a bad haircut, it grows out. If you lose a fingernail, it grows back. If you cut your finger or scratch your eye, it heals. Not your enamel. Every insult is sustained for a lifetime. Why?

Then one day the answer dawned on me. It's because the teeth of a *healthy* human are designed to last your whole life. Teeth shouldn't dissolve or decay ... ever!

Sadly, that's not the world we now live in. Consider yourself very unusual if your child hasn't had a cavity by the fourth grade. Today, almost 20% of our two-year-olds and one-third of our three-year-olds already have tooth decay in process. Half of all kids have at least one cavity filled by midchildhood and 80% by late adolescence! But it's just a cavity, right? It's so common we seem to think nothing of it. After all, that's why we go to the dentist, right? To find out how many cavities we have? Hmmm.

Here's where I need to pause to give you a full admission. I really wrestled with the subtitle of this book. Raising Healthy Happy Kids ... *Against All Odds*? I wondered if I'd offend you by telling you, right up front, that the odds are your child will *not* grow up healthy. Unfortunately, I can make that claim by looking at kids' *teeth*, alone!

It's a tragic situation, really. These days, your hospital's surgical department has an unending lineup of toddlers scheduled to be sedated, under general anesthesia, to have a bunch of dental extractions and major restorations (crowns) for a mouthful of bombed-out teeth.

This has been a continually progressing problem throughout post-industrialized society. In the late 1930s, a brilliant dentist and nutritionist, Dr. Weston A. Price, exposed the significance of dental damage *and* malocclusion (smaller faces with crowded teeth) due to a carbohydrate-heavy, Westernized diet. He compared this new phenomenon to those populations of people who were consuming *no* industrialized foods, where he documented the near absence of cavities or malocclusion!

Today, the resulting dental disease is a bigger catastrophe than you can possibly imagine. Affecting more than half of the world's population, caries disease (the disease of tooth decay) is the *number one most prevalent* of all 291 diseases included in the Global Burden of Disease Study. And early childhood caries disease (cavities under six years old) is the number one most prevalent disease amongst young children ... *worldwide*!

Now that I have your attention, here's what every Brave Parent needs to know. *Caries disease is 100% preventable!* We just need to change a few risk factors during the first year of life. Just ahead you'll learn more about those risk factors in section 7.4 Early Childhood Caries Disease.

"

Tooth enamel is unlike the other part of our body's **ectoderm** (the body's outer covering that includes skin, hair, nails, and cornea of the eye). Enamel **doesn't repair itself** following injury or disease! That means, if you get a bad haircut, it grows out. If you lose a fingernail, it grows back. If you cut your finger or scratch your eye, it heals. **Not your enamel.** Every insult is sustained for a **lifetime.**

Why?

It's because the teeth of a **healthy human** are designed to **last your whole life.** Teeth shouldn't dissolve or decay ... **ever!**

"

There are primarily four oral diseases that can steal your teeth, and every one of these is on the rise today:

- *Caries disease* (tooth decay)
- *Periodontal disease* (infection in the gums and bone support)
- *Occlusal disease* (chipped, cracked, and worn-down teeth from clenching and grinding)
- *Oropharyngeal cancer* (primarily caused by HPV from oral sex and steals more than your teeth)

It probably comes as no surprise that the prevalence of oral diseases is climbing right along with our other lifestyle-related diseases. Each of these is complex in nature. I will explore all four and discuss how we can get kids on track to maintain super healthy teeth and gums for a lifetime—starting in the first year of life.

By the way, in case you think information on oropharyngeal cancer from sexually transmitted infections doesn't belong in a book on pediatric health, I have to break the bad news. Up to 24% of ten- to thirteen-year-olds and 33–59% of high school teens report that they have either given or received oral sex.

So, brace yourself, because this chapter is going to take you on a ride you probably didn't expect when considering your kiddo's oral health.

7.1 INFANT ORAL HEALTH EXAM

Until about 2010, three years old was considered the most appropriate age for a first-time dental visit. But in the last decade we've been enlightened by a new paradigm. Today, health professionals who see kids at least *know* about the American Academy of Pediatric Dentistry (AAPD) recommendation—babies should be examined in their new "dental home" (their identified dental office) *under the age of one!* Specifically, between the eruption of their first tooth (about six months old) and before their first birthday. Again, I promise to tell you why we've zoomed in on this specific window of time when we get to section 7.4 on caries disease prevention.

Most family docs and pediatricians got the memo and have added "infant oral health examination" to their routine checklist of parent to-dos. Unfortunately, general dentists are lagging behind. If you call your family dentist to request an exam for your infant, don't be surprised if the receptionist tells you they don't see children until the age of three. Or maybe they'll invite your child to accompany you next time, to get a free ride in the dental chair.

I suppose dentists are resistant to change because most didn't learn to examine babies in dental school. And frankly, with the exception of pediatric dentists, most of my profession don't understand *why* the recommendation changed in the first place, or *what* to do during that appointment.

In addition to a deep dive into caries disease prevention strategies, the checklist of topics we cover includes a thorough assessment of:

- Importance of 24/7 nasal breathing (see chapter 4 Breathe)
- Quality and quantity of sleep (see chapter 5 Sleep)
- Nutrition (including the Food Rules in chapter 1 Eat and chapter 3 Digest)
- Establishing good food relationships (see chapter 1 Eat)
- Oral-facial growth and development (see chapter 4 Breathe)
- Swallowing (see section 4.15 on Myofunctional Therapy in chapter 4 Breathe)
- Dental safety at home and play, including what to do in an emergency
- Nonnutritive sucking habits, such as finger, thumb, and pacifier (see chapter 4 Breathe)

66

Today, the resulting **dental disease** is a bigger **catastrophe** than you can possibly imagine. Affecting more than half of the world's population, **caries disease** (the disease of *tooth decay*) is the number one **most prevalent** of all 291 diseases included in the Global Burden of Disease Study. And early childhood caries disease (cavities under six years old) is the **number one most prevalent disease** amongst young children ... worldwide!

Now that I have your attention, here's what every *Brave Parent* needs to know. Caries disease is **100% preventable!** We just need to change a few risk factors during the first year of life.

99

In my office, most of this one-hour infant appointment is an educational dialogue with the Registered Dental Hygienist. In fact, the only part that physically involves the baby is the "knee-to-knee exam." In a sitting position, the parent's knees are against mine, and the baby, in a hugging position with mom or dad, leans back to rest their head on my lap. Within a minute or two, I can examine their mouth, tongue, airway (posterior pharynx), tonsils, nostrils, and teeth, of course. Then with a swipe of fluoride varnish on their newly erupted teeth, the baby's job is done.

The AAPD and ADA recommend six-month preventive visits going forward.

7.2 ENFORCING GOOD EATS

During the infant oral health exam, I always emphasize how important the infant and toddler years are in establishing healthy eating behaviors. This is a continual challenge because *parents become the teachers*, but they're often not eating healthily themselves. I've noticed that there's never a time when adults are more curious about what it takes to establish a healthier lifestyle than when they're pregnant or beginning to care for a baby. They're very open to establishing better eating habits. They just need guidance.

It bears repeating that good food is nature's remedy for almost everything! A wide variety of nutrients act as the building blocks for all cell health, including dental health. Keep in mind that *all* disease begins at the cellular level, and your child's ability to fend off illness depends on their daily intake of *phytonutrients* (plant-based elements that are integral to proper cell function).

Even during infancy, when babies might be getting their primary nutrients from breastmilk, it's critically important for you, Brave Parents, to establish a plan that will turn your child's diet in the *opposite direction* from most American children.

Review the chapters on Eat, Drink, and Digest from time to time, where you'll rediscover what you need to update your plan, including helping your growing child develop a healthy relationship to food, establishing a low-sugar, fiber-rich, nutrient-dense diet, and tips for avoiding processed, commercial foods and drinks. Also feel free to share the two-page synopsis of Dr. Susan's Food Pillars with your friends and family. You'll find a downloadable pdf on the BeABraveParent.com website.

7.3 AVOIDING ENAMEL DEFECTS

By the time I'd had Hunter, I'd grown curious about why I was seeing so many of my little patients' teeth erupt with developmental flaws in their enamel. Most often these are caused by a significant illness or high fever that the child suffered during the calcification process, long before the tooth erupted. But I saw lots of yellow- and white-spot defects with no traceable cause, and I was convinced they had something to do with food additives.

I studied the FDA's GRAS list (food additives that are Generally Recognized as Safe), and it looks *anything but safe* to me! Being a tooth-fanatical nerd, I simply avoided feeding my child commercial foods with additives. I never got a great answer to our developmental defect phenomenon, but I remain skeptical. Meanwhile, Hunter reaped a thousand other inadvertent benefits from avoiding processed food during his "little" years. At twenty-eight, he still has beautiful, strong, filling-free teeth and a lean, robust, healthy body to boot.

7.4 EARLY CHILDHOOD CARIES DISEASE (ECC), THE DISEASE OF TOOTH DECAY

Our world can't seem to get a handle on this epidemic of toddler tooth decay. We saw a whopping 38% increase in decay rates for two- to five-year-olds between the years 1999 and 2004! It won't turn around until we (1) get control of the sugary drink obsession and (2) think about it like the transmissible bacterial infection it is. That will require a paradigm shift even among dental professionals and Brave Parents alike.

Most of us, likely including your dental health professionals, assume that the way to fix tooth decay is to allow the dentist to drill into the tooth, clean out the decay, and fill the remaining hole with a nonnatural tooth substitute, such as composite resin. That is clearly *not* the case. It's true that drilling and filling the tooth is how we fix the hole *created* by the decay, but it has nothing to do with remedying the caries disease itself.

> **"**
>
> Most of us, likely including your *dental health* professionals, assume that the way to **fix tooth decay** is to allow the dentist to **drill** into the tooth, clean out the decay, and fill the remaining hole with a **non-natural** tooth substitute, such as composite **resin.**
>
> That is clearly *not* the case."
>
> **"**

Here's my best analogy. If you drove home to find your house engulfed in flames, would you call a carpenter to fix the roof while the fire was still licking away at your floorboards? Of course not! You'd call 911 to summon the fire department, who'd soon show up and wrestle that destructive fire to a halt! Next, the authorities would identify the *cause* of the fire—you'd definitely want to fix that in order to prevent a future fire. And finally, you'd get a restorative plan in place for the reconstruction ... including the roof.

My profession usually does it backward. When your dentist detects a couple cavities at your so-called preventive appointment, you schedule another appointment to drill and fill. Meanwhile, we stand by as the caries disease that caused the holes smolders on.

There is another way! If you've been haunted by ongoing dental decay (active caries disease) throughout your life, ask your dentist or hygienist for time to talk, not drill. Let them help you tease out your contributing influences from among the *many* identified risk factors. Let's take a look at what those might be.

My cavity-prone patients often say something like this: "It's always been this way. I just inherited bad teeth." And I like to answer, "It's much more likely that you inherited bad bugs!" As we discussed in chapter 3 Digest, we are born with a relatively sterile mouth (and gut), but on our way into the world through the birth canal, we get a mouthful of mom's vaginal and gut bacterial strains, and immediately after, her skin bacterial strains from breastfeeding. But mom's saliva contains another huge ration of bugs—both helpful and harmful.

Adults' mouths are a home to hundreds of identifiable bacterial strains, which can inadvertently be transferred to a baby's mouth through a single drop of saliva ... from a spoon, cup, pacifier, juicy kiss, or licked index finger that swoops in to clean up a baby's mouth.

In that way, mom or dad (or *any* primary caregiver) can inoculate your baby's mouth with a sizable dose of one or two of the most significant acid-producing bacterial strains, Streptococcus mutans and Lactobacillus acidophilus. The population size of these transferred bugs appears to influence your kiddo's cavity-proneness forever. There is a higher risk of disease severity (meaning a higher cavity rate) if the spit-swapping caregiver is cavity-prone!

At this time, the science supports the concept of a *window of infectivity.* That is, if you can avoid saliva transmission *before* the eruption of your baby's first molars (about one year old) to about three and a half years old, you will help your kiddo avoid decay for the rest of their life.

If you want the nitty gritty, it's because the biggest acid-producing bug strains recognize the deep grooves of your kiddos first molars as a nice new home. They settle in, unpack their bags, and multiply. So as long as we quell the spit-swap before the first molar erupts (on average at age one), you're good!

> "At this time, the science *supports* the concept of a window of infectivity. That is, if you can **avoid saliva transmission** before the eruption of your **baby's first molars** (about one year old) to about three and a half years old, you will help your kiddo *avoid decay* for the rest of their life."

Practically speaking that means truly avoiding mouth kisses, sharing spoons or cups, using a wet finger to clean your baby's mouth, sucking on a fallen pacifier before you give it back, and other seemingly innocent mistakes.

This might be astonishing news for you, your friends, or family, so help spread the word to *all* your baby's caregivers. Meanwhile, in a world where most parents (and grands) miss the memo, and these cavity-forming bugs are insidiously pervasive in our population, most babies don't get a pass. So, let's focus next on what brave efforts you can make *beyond* avoiding transmission.

7.5 HOW CAVITIES ARE FORMED

Turns out, those acid-secreting bugs *love* sugar—even more than we do! They gobble it up, metabolize it, and spit out *acid* as a by-product.

You can explain it to kiddos like this: "These teeny-tiny bugs eat SUGAR and then *pee* on your teeth! That's yucky! So, our goal is *not to feed the bugs!*" That explanation usually rouses wide eyes and giggles, but it also seems to gross them out.

As far as teeth are concerned, it's not the concentration of sugar or the amount of sugar you provide the bugs but the *frequency.* You see, once the bugs feast and pee, your saliva neutralizes the acid in about a half hour. But if you're a sweet-drink sipper (versus a slugger), or if you've become a candy nibbler throughout the day, these bugs live like little kings and queens, gorging on a constant source of sugar. And your teeth will pay the price.

Tooth decay progresses from the outside in. With an ongoing supply of sweet foods and drinks, the sugar-loving cavity bugs flourish. They keep spitting acid until they create a decalcified *white spot* on the enamel. It can happen as quickly as six weeks in a low pH (high acid) environment.

Next, the white spot caves in to a little divot. (Incidentally, the word *cavity* shares a root with the word *cave.* It's derived from the Latin word *cavus,* which means *hollow.*)

The divot serves as a protective bungalow for the sugar-loving bacteria, and once their whole bug party moves into this "cave," the critters become protected from a toothbrush and floss. Lucky them ... and unlucky us!

Straightaway, the sugar-bug invasion progresses to the inner layer of tooth structure called *dentin*. Because dentin is seven times softer than enamel, the bugs can run like wildfire, and *boom!* ... we have a full-blown cavity.

7.6 CAVITY DETECTION IN THE DENTAL OFFICE

Because acid-spitting bugs hang out en masse within the plaque layer, we see *patterns* of destruction in the teeth wherever the plaque is heaviest. For example, your child's dentist might show you cavities between teeth in the X-rays, just below the place where side-by-side teeth contact each other. Or the decay might be in the grooves of the biting surfaces, or even at the gumline on cheek-side surfaces.

If your child is diagnosed with decay, I encourage you to ask your dentist and hygienist for a good look at your child's cavities, including any white spots (beginning cavities) too. A picture is worth a thousand words, and fantastic and giant images are right at our fingertips through the use of intraoral photographs and digital cavity-detecting X-rays (called bitewings).

Looking at the images, ask your dentist to help you understand the criteria she's using about what to fill and what to "observe for now." All of this gives you a better understanding of your child's disease patterns and how to help put out the fire.

With a little explanation, reading high-tech digital X-rays on a big screen is easy. I recently described to Carlos, a five-year-old boy, how I can "see" when his cavity extends beyond the enamel layer into the dentin—that's the criteria I use to determine whether it needs to be drilled and filled now or if it can be postponed for observation on next year's X-rays. Then I flashed through images of all five of Carlos's cavities, and to my delight, he diagnosed each one of them with 100% accuracy. Two needed fillings, and three were to be observed.

Later that evening I received a glowing email from Carlos's mom, saying that he boasted to his dad that evening, "I know I have five cavities, but Dr. Susan told me I was the very best five-year-old X-ray reader in the whole world!" I hit reply and, with a wink-face emoji, reminded her that Carlos has ZERO competition.

When you're informed your kiddo has decay, it's a good time to ask the dentist's or hygienist's opinion on how best to stabilize it. Remember to always ask questions in front of your child, so they can *own their disease* and hear what it will take to secure a healthier future.

Attention Brave Parents, if you are consistent in your messaging, it can absolutely damper their sweet-snacking, sugar-sipping desires. After all, no one wants cavities!

Here's a funny story: When my son was about six years old, my psychologist mama faulted me for making her grandson overly anxious about getting cavities. Full disclosure: Hunter had already had two little cavities filled in his baby teeth and decidedly, did not want another. Apparently, while spending the night at Grama's house, he finished brushing his teeth and asked for her help with flossing. She said, "Well, I must've given him a funny look because he immediately said with a sigh, 'I can tell you really don't want to, Grama. It's okay if we don't floss *all* of them tonight, but at least I want to floss the tight contacts and two beginning cavities. C'mon, I'll show you where they are.'"

Maybe she was right, but the proof is in the pudding. Hunter's two old fillings went to the tooth fairy, and he never had another cavity.

I encourage you to schedule six-month visits to your child's dentist, while you do regular visual inspections at home too. Don't wait till your child has a discomfort to get help. Even though baby teeth are a practice set, they need to be filled before the decay reaches the inner "pulp" chamber and begins to inflict pain. By then, the tooth usually requires extraction.

7.7 EXTRACTION

As caries disease advances, deep cavities can affect pulp health. Dying teeth can cause excruciating pain and infection (also known as an abscess), gum swelling, facial swelling, and more. While pulp death in adult teeth can usually be remedied by root canal therapy, we are not as successful with our heroic efforts to save sick baby teeth, so we lean toward extraction. Luckily a new healthy tooth will eventually take its place.

You can breathe a sigh of relief at the loss of an abscessed tooth, but beware! Without the baby tooth as a placeholder, the adjacent teeth can drift into the new space, hindering the eruption of its permanent replacement tooth. So, your dentist will likely recommend placing a mini orthodontic retainer called a *space maintainer* until the permanent tooth erupts.

I don't want to oversimplify caries disease. For adults it can be very challenging to tease out the many contributing factors that may underly your active decay. Anything that helps create an acidic environment are added risk factors.

Let's start with acid reflux—because 60% of our population have it occasionally and 30% have it weekly. This common ailment can be rooted in food sensitivities, chemical food additives, and sleep-disordered breathing. (Refer back to the Eat, Breathe, and Sleep chapters.) But for now, recognize that a single drop of stomach acid that enters the throat and mouth drastically increases mouth acidity.

Other common factors are dry mouth (from medications, cannabis, alcohol, or tobacco, for example), eating or drinking acidic drinks (like coffee, soda, lemon water, and some bottled waters), eating acidic foods which are almost any processed food from a jar or a can. Late-night carb snacking is an issue also, as saliva stops flowing at night, so your bedtime acid level persists through the long hours of the night.

This is the same reason infants can get *baby bottle tooth decay*, a.k.a. *bottle rot*. If your baby falls asleep while eating, the sugar in formula or breast milk will feed the cavity bugs all night long. So once your baby has erupted teeth, it's best to feed him or her an hour before bedtime, if at all possible.

To help support your children in avoiding this bug-feeding frenzy, eliminate all sugary beverages (including juice), candy, fruit snacks, and sweetened breakfast cereals from your grocery cart.

For the latest science on caries disease, I highly recommend Dr. Kim Kutsch's new book, *Why Me?* Dr. Kutsch is not only the author, but the founder of CariFree, arguably the best resource for products to help you effectively put out the fire.

7.8 WHAT'S FLUORIDE ALL ABOUT?

In the early 1900s, as we industrialized our food supply, sugar consumption climbed in the US, and so did the cavity rate. That should have been a good indication that we really needed to dial back on our sugar consumption. But, NO! In our shortsightedness, we instead hunted for a Band-Aid to cover up the problem. And we found it.

A young dentist, Dr. Frederick McKay spent thirty years tracking down the natural ingredient that made the teeth of early twentieth-century residents of Colorado Springs so resistant to decay. You already know the answer—fluoride. Then in 1945, trying to ratchet down the ever-growing decay rate, the US began a massive effort to add fluoride to our drinking water.

Today, about 73% of our municipal water systems have added fluoride, specifically to bind to the tooth structure before your kiddo's teeth ever erupt. It seems that fluoride used in this way is considered a drug, according to the Food and Drug Administration. And not all the people receiving that treatment necessarily agree to it. But pediatricians and dentists agree that we don't want you to miss this window of opportunity to strengthen your kids' teeth for a lifetime.

Thus, the fluoride controversy drags on and on ... and I get it. Let me talk more about how and why the fluoride molecule works, and whether we think it should be here to stay.

But first, let's get this much straight. It is not an inherent lack of fluoride in (or on) our teeth that is causing our ever-increasing decay rate! Unfortunately, since we, as a culture, seem entirely unwilling to dial back our sugar consumption, and food manufactures won't do it for us, fluoride remains the gold standard for protecting enamel.

There are two very different ways the fluoride molecule defends a tooth. First from the inside, layering into developing enamel as a building-block for lifelong protection. That's called systemic fluoride. And second, by fortifying the outside surface of the enamel, after a tooth has already been formed and erupted. That's called topical fluoride.

7.9 SYSTEMIC FLUORIDE

It's true that systemic fluoride exposure during their years of growth and development (from birth till age twelve) creates an inherently stronger, more cavity-resistant protective layer than natural enamel. The result: a 40% to 60% lifetime protection from decay, according to a study in the *Journal of Public Health Dentistry*.

Although many developed countries do not add fluoride to their water supplies, in the United States some 73% of water systems add fluoride salt, also known as sodium fluoride, in concentrations less than one part per million. The EPA regulates the amount in accordance with the Safe Drinking Water Act. At such low dosages, fluoride strengthens teeth without proven potential for negative health effects. That said, all you have to do is google "negative effects of fluoride in water" to see the barrage of controversial thoughts about the possible health threats from fluoridated water. Concerns are based on everything from legitimate scientific research to freedom of choice issues and even government conspiracy theories.

Personally, I wish we didn't have the need to add *anything* to our drinking water. But I have not seen enough quality evidence around health threats from systemic fluoride to outweigh the enormous body of science supporting tooth protection in a world where tooth decay is our most prevalent disease. As I'm a dentist for people of all ages, I have a keen eye on health benefits from keeping your kiddo's teeth intact for their lifetime! So, please don't shoot me if you're on the other side of this controversy. In truth, and for the record, I'm a much bigger fan of getting control of our sugared-up processed food consumption than fluoridating our water. But when's that going to happen?

If you want fluoride protection for your child and you don't live in an area with access to a fluoridated water system, you will want to have your water tested. Most county health departments offer water analysis at no or low cost. Take the sample from your kitchen sink where most of your cooking and drinking water comes from. Then share the results with your dentist, who will determine if your child needs a fluoride supplement—and the precise amount, based on their age and body weight. I want to stress the importance of a professionally calculated prescription because too much fluoride causes a condition called fluorosis, marked by permanent brown spots in the enamel. On average I prescribe about .1 milligram a day for kids who have no fluoride in water at home or school and half that for those who drink fluoridated drinking water while at school.

Dentists have historically believed that systemic fluoride is more beneficial than topical fluoride (used on the surface of teeth). But the dental literature keeps flip-flopping on which is best. With the surge of sugar consumption and increased acidity in our food supply, topical application seems to be winning. I recommend both.

" Let's get this much *straight.*

It is not an inherent **lack of fluoride** in (or on) our teeth that is causing our **ever-increasing decay rate!** Unfortunately, since we, as a culture, seem entirely unwilling to dial back our **sugar consumption**, and food manufactures won't do it for us, fluoride remains the

gold standard

for **protecting enamel. "**

7.10 TOPICAL FLUORIDE

Your tooth enamel is made up of tiny rods that are perpendicular to the surface of your tooth. Similar to the pores of your skin, these rods suck up fluids. So, when you apply topical fluoride, it soaks into your tooth—although this protectant must be continually replenished throughout life to be most effective.

Here's an experiment we do in our children's Hands-On Learning Lab™ that helps my kiddos learn about the effectiveness of topical fluoride. We start by soaking an egg in a sodium fluoride solution for five to ten minutes. Then we transfer it to a beaker of clear acid—either a brand-name lemon-lime soda or white vinegar. In the "control" beaker, we drop an *untreated* egg into the liquid acid and watch the action. The surface of the natural eggshell immediately begins to bubble up and fizz. Over time the acid destroys the entire shell. But the fluoride-soaked egg ... just sits like an impenetrable rock! Boring to watch, the fluoride absorption keeps the egg completely protected.

So how do we get topical fluoride? Tap water is one source, albeit a weak one. Commercial toothpastes and over-the-counter rinses are another. But far more effective sources are applied professionally every three to six months. These treatments are called fluoride varnish. They dry quickly and will set even in the presence of saliva, so there's less gagging and swallowing than with the gooey gels and icky foams you endured in your childhood. Applying varnish is as simple as a quick swipe with a little paintbrush. Up-to-date pediatricians are even swooshing it on during the annual well-child visit.

Cavity-prone kids and adults can benefit from daily topical exposure with higher concentration, prescription-based products. Your best bet for a cavity-prone kid is to talk with your dentist to develop a personalized fluoride protection plan.

> 66 The idea of leaving the dentist without having your teeth polished is just bizarre to most people. We're *creatures of habit.* The only reason your children (or **YOU**) should have those pearly whites polished is ... to **remove stain, and stain alone**! (In case you're wondering, stain on teeth is **not harmful,** it's just ugly.)" 99

7.11 THE NEWEST RECOMMENDATIONS IN TOOTHPASTES FOR INFANTS

Since there is a scant amount of fluoride in most toothpastes, and we want to avoid overexposure, we have historically recommended that little ones avoid these until they're able to spit (versus swallow) after brushing. Now we recommend that littles (ages one to three) use the fluoride toothpaste but only matching the size of a grain of rice.

Toothpastes taste sweet and can be appealing to a child, especially if you're braving it out with a juice-free, candy-free home. I remember seeing my BFFs sugar-deprived kiddos heaping on the toothpaste and making *yummy* sounds as they haphazardly swallowed it. I alarmedly told Vicki her kids were *eating* the toothpaste as a bedtime snack and advised her to take them out for ice cream once in a while. We had a good laugh. Incidentally, all three of these kids grew up cavity free, and all three of them, Anthony, Nichole, and Ashlynn, are orthodontists/dentists today. Furthermore, they are all touting the benefits of growing up sugar-robbed, daily exercisers, and uber healthy ... *against all odds*!

7.12 SELECTIVE POLISHING

This is probably the best time to mention a well-documented concept that every dentist and hygienist learns in dental school: *selective polishing*—polishing teeth with a rubber cup and pumice paste is not so good for our enamel. It's particularly harmful to baby teeth, as the polish abrades the fluoride-rich enamel surface that we have built up over repeated applications. Furthermore, the tooth's natural biofilm layer acts as a scaffold for the fluoride varnish to stay put and keep absorbing into the tooth surface for several hours after application.

The idea of leaving the dentist without having your teeth polished is just bizarre to most people. We're creatures of habit. The only reason your children (or YOU) should have those pearly whites polished is ... to remove stain, and stain alone! (In case you're wondering, stain on teeth is not harmful, it's just ugly.)

Instead of polishing, I'm a big proponent of the *self-prophy*, a.k.a. the *toothbrush prophy*, where children learn how to effectively remove their own plaque, every day, not just when they visit the dentist. This follows the parable: Give a man a fish and you feed him for a day; teach a man to fish and you feed him for a lifetime. I will explain self-prophy in much more detail under the Oral Hygiene and Skill-Building sections in this chapter.

Meanwhile, when I challenge audiences of my colleagues about why they still haven't ditched their outmoded practices of polishing teeth, they usually tell me they do it to manage their patients' expectations. They think everyone wants to leave with that silky, smooth, naked-enamel feel. It lasts only for about thirty minutes.

I have to remind them that many kids and adults today are *not* leaving us with the slick feel of pumiced teeth, rather the rough, sandpaper feel of fluoride varnish ... and that the varnish works even better on teeth that haven't been polished with pumice.

Topical fluoride has taken on another important role for children and adults alike, protecting our teeth from acid erosion. Our commercialized, processed food diets have become much more acidic than ever. Think of drinks alone. All the juices, sports drinks, sodas, and diet sodas we guzzle have a pH (a measure of acidity) hundreds of times more than that of plain water.

For children and adults, fluoride varnish also desensitizes teeth. It slows down the metabolism of bacteria that cause cavities. And finally, it reduces the number of the cavity-causing bacteria, *Streptococcus mutans*, by more than tenfold.

7.13 PREVENTING GUM DISEASE

For adults, the other wildly pervasive oral disease is *periodontal disease (PD)*, where the supporting structures around the tooth become either inflamed, infected, or both. By thirty years old, *half* of us have active PD that, in many ways, threatens the life of the tooth *and*, rather significantly, the systemic health of the host.

It seems like yesterday—only a couple decades ago—when we were still telling our patients that this chronic bacterial infection was no threat to our overall health, only to hanging on to our teeth. It's true that PD causes the gums to unzip, the bone to melt away, the teeth to drift, and then eventually to fall out.

But oh, how the plot has thickened. Our research-based paradigm has shifted, linking periodontal disease to fifty-seven different systemic diseases. And as recently as 2016, PD was proven to *cause* heart attack and stroke.

Historically, my profession blamed the patient for their disease, putting most of our emphasis on their lack of effective oral hygiene. We seriously *believed* PD was mostly due to a lack of daily plaque removal, and since we typically see more bone loss between teeth, we told patients it was mainly caused by their failure to floss. Don't get me wrong. Your daily plaque "disruption" is a significant factor in maintaining (or recreating) healthy gums and bone. But it's not that simple.

It's a complicated, multi-factorial disease but it boils down to two significant challenges. One, maintaining (or recreating) a healthy microbial biofilm. That is, reducing the concentrations of dangerous bugs that grow on and around your gumline. Two, maintaining (or recreating) a strong host resistance to these bad bugs. That means putting your body in a position of optimal health. Both of these are much easier said than done!

We still gauge periodontal disease activity with a hand instrument—a pocket-measuring probe—which measures not only pocket depths but whether the disease is currently *active*, meaning inflamed. Gums that bleed right after probing, brushing, or flossing is a sure sign of active inflammation. So is puffiness and redness.

Today our sophistication around a solid approach to treating this bacteria-induced infection relies heavily on our pregame analysis. I now rely on laboratory analysis of saliva for the identification of specific dangerous bacterial strains and the corresponding antibiotic(s) that might be necessary to shift the microbiome of the diseased mouth.

We also use a fingerstick blood test for detection of huge blood sugar levels (undiagnosed or uncontrolled diabetes). If suspected, we use saliva to identify any of nine fungal (candida) infections we might suspect. Beyond that, we must consider the potential role of food sensitivities (such as gluten, dairy, or nightshades), diet/nutrient deficiencies, saliva dysfunction (dry mouth), smoking, and many other personal health/autoimmune challenges.

After gathering all the data, we can design a personalized strategy to treat and stabilize the disease effectively. It's never simple, however. And without gathering and addressing data, we seem to keep people in what I call the *perio-go-round*, watching it flair up again and again throughout their lifetime.

Periodontal disease is generally an adult disease, and as you might have already guessed, it is 100% *preventable*. So, let's turn our attention to preventing PD in children. That means focusing on mastering self-care—both in terms of oral hygiene and establishing nutritional and other lifestyle habits that predict a lifetime of optimal health.

7.14 ORAL HYGIENE

Since oral home care is a critical element for preventing caries and periodontal disease, fostering your kiddo's ongoing progression of daily home-care habits has a big payoff. Even before your baby's teeth erupt (about six months of age), it's wise to begin to stimulate his/her mouth by wiping the gums with a clean, damp washcloth. And as the first teeth erupt, you can introduce a soft brush for daily cleaning. This might be old news for you, but what's new is our toothpaste recommendation.

Fostering your kiddo's ongoing progression of **daily home-care habits** has a

big payoff.

Even before your baby's teeth erupt (about six months of age), it's wise to begin to stimulate his/her mouth by

wiping the gums

with a clean, damp washcloth.

And as the **first teeth erupt**, you can introduce a

soft brush

for **daily cleaning.**

Until 2014 we recommended using a small dab of fluoride-free toothpaste, reserving fluoride until your child was able to spit out (rather than swallow) the residual toothpaste. Then in 2014, responding to the continual rise in ECC (decay), the American Academy of Pediatrics made an official recommendation to start babies with a small "smear" of fluoridated toothpaste as soon as the first teeth erupt. The element of fluoride, absorbed topically into the outside of the tooth, truly helps strengthen the enamel, so it better resists decay over the lifetime of the tooth.

7.15 EARLY SKILL-BUILDING

As children grow in their hand coordination, they can assist in their own self-care. But until a child can demonstrate the ability to clean the entire mouth thoroughly, a parent needs to finish the job.

As a dentist, I have a goal for every child, by the age of eighteen, to develop *skills, beliefs, and habits* for a lifetime of oral and *systemic* health. If we achieve this, along with a practiced understanding of how diet plays a critical role, we will see children avoid a mouthful of cavities and gum disease and keep their strong teeth for a lifetime.

For special needs children, most or all of the responsibility will rest on caregivers, perhaps always. In order to avoid severe dental disease in kids who aren't able to chew and swallow fibrous foods, maintaining good daily home care and avoiding sugar becomes even more important.

In choosing a dentist and dental hygienist for your kiddo, look for a partnership, someone willing to invest in a personal relation-ship with your child (and you) that fosters your child's progress toward self-care and optimal health.

Many parents are curious about what kind of toothbrush and floss we recommend, and the answer is ... whatever works. I want children to know how to use *all* the available over-the-counter prod-ucts—properly! For example, a battery-driven power brush is far and away more efficient and effective than a handheld brush (according to every comparative study), even though a traditional handheld brush can definitely be used effectively.

Just remember the proper techniques are vastly different, and children need to be coached in their skill development for each. A traditional brush requires proper placement and brushing hand movement, whereas the power brush just requires placement. Dragging the brush creepy-slow along the gumline does the trick. Because it takes so much less coordination, this is especially beneficial for young children and geriatric patients, who might develop diminishing motor skills. That said, my entire dental team also uses a power brush daily.

7.16 A NEW PARADIGM FOR TEACHING SELF-CARE

For the first fifteen years of my dental practice, the dental hygiene part of a child's visit (called the *prophy*, short for prophylaxis) was quite conventional. We polished their teeth, demonstrated toothbrushing on a model, tossed a new toothbrush in a take-home goodie bag, and called it a day. The problem was it didn't work. Sure, we *talked* about health, but we were definitely not fostering the skills, habitual behaviors, or beliefs to support our words.

Perplexed by this problem, I discovered this proverb by a Confucian scholar named Xunzi:

I hear and I forget.

I see and I remember.

I do and I understand.

With the help of my dedicated team members, we transformed our traditional hygiene visit into a completely nonconventional approach—and it's one you can do at home. Rather than performing the cleaning for them, we support each child in accomplishing *their own* thorough cleaning.

We swab their teeth with "2Tone" disclosing solution. It stains their dental plaque pink and purple. The two colors reveal *old plaque* (the stuff that's been undisrupted for more than twenty-four hours) and *new plaque* (missed for less than twenty-four hours). After a good inspection in a lighted mirror, it's time to go to work. Each kiddo *chooses*, from a grand array of tooth cleaning devices, what they would like to use to clean the colored plaque off their teeth.

Engaging in *choice* accomplishes two things. First, we can teach them, over years, how to effectively use *each* invention of toothbrush, power brush, pointed brush, string floss, and floss gadget. Second, and perhaps most important, the very act of choosing instills *a more personal interest and sense of engagement.* I want them to go home from each and every visit with a renewed excitement in their new skill development.

We call this individualized, mentored approach to self-care a *self-prophy.*

In the clinical notes, we track their progress, capabilities, barriers, and specified goals. Our mission is to take each child one step further toward a lifetime of health with each and every visit.

When a child is in an active learning phase, it's sometimes beneficial to increase their self-prophy frequency, even to once a week or once a month. More frequent visits are especially helpful for any kiddo with physical or mental challenges that impede our goal—*to establish beliefs, skills, and habits for a lifetime of oral health.*

I mentioned that you can do a self-prophy at home. Here's how. Just buy some Gum Red-Cote disclosing tablets and have them chew one, swish, and spit. It will paint their plaque red. Then be fully present and encouraging while your child goes to work to brush and floss away what they've missed. Stay particularly attentive to your child's *individual* abilities for self-care, and take them one step further, time after time. And don't forget to celebrate their progress.

66 I mentioned that you can do a **self-prophy at home.** Here's how. Just buy some **Gum Red-Cote** disclosing tablets and have them chew one, swish, and spit. It will **paint their plaque red.** Then be fully present and encouraging while your child goes to work to

brush and floss

away what they've missed. Stay particularly attentive to your child's individual abilities for **self-care**, and take them one step further, time after time. And don't forget to **celebrate their progress.** 99

7.17 TOOTH GRINDING AT NIGHT (A.K.A. SLEEP BRUXISM)

Many parents ask me about why their kids grind their teeth at night, and my answers have varied over my years in practice. Not because I'm wishy-washy, but because my information is continually changing. The truth is, grinding noises during sleep are fairly common in children—but once again, common doesn't mean healthy. The science supports a variety of causes.

Flashback! I remember a time when pinworms were one of the biggest risk factors for pediatric sleep bruxism. Even today, pinworm infection ranges from .2% to 20% of our kid population, depending on where you live. When the worms poke their heads out of a child's poop-shoot at night to lay their eggs, it stimulates teeth gnashing. (Sounds fitting, doesn't it?) Trust me, it wasn't fun being the dentist who convinced parents to collect proof (pinworm eggs) by spreading their kiddos' butt cheeks and dabbing a piece of masking tape on their bungholes ... while they slept.

These days, when I'm asked about sleep bruxism, I think of airway deficiencies first. Recall in the chapters on Breathe and Sleep, I described at length the crowded pharynx and compromised tongue box situation. Now picture how a sleeping child, on either end of REM sleep, can benefit from sliding the lower jaw forward and/or sideways to open up more room for the tongue to get out of the throat. Tooth grinding for airway obstructions, even in adults, helps support 24/7 nasal breathing, but at the expense of our precious, irreplicable tooth structure.

Some children brux because they have early childhood malocclusion (ECM), and during their unconscious hours, they are trying to grind out interferences and grind in a better chewing position.

Other common reasons for night grinding are stress, anxiety, and chronic pain. These ailments can benefit from regular relaxation practices such as mindfulness-based stress reduction (MBSR). See chapter 6 Feel and Think for more on this.

When tooth grinding degrades baby teeth, we get less excited since this "practice set" goes to the tooth fairy. But we want to find the root cause and address it before we replicate the damage in the permanent teeth.

Along the way, a few of my little grinders develop symptoms such as tooth sensitivity, painful chewing, sore muscles, or jaw joint (TMJ) pain. While I can usually remedy these issues in adults with a precision-made "bite splint" or a sleep appliance to be worn regularly at nighttime, that's not a workable solution for growing kids. Consult your dentist to see if he or she can make a temporary splint, as these acute symptoms will usually subside in a matter of days.

7.18 WHAT TO EXPECT FROM YOUR ORTHODONTIST

Everyone loves a pretty smile! We have developed a cultural bias toward straight, white teeth and an ear-to-ear toothy smile. Most people don't get so lucky on their own. Today over four million people in the US are wearing braces at any one time, and 75% of them are children.

It's reported that 70–80% of our population has dental crowding. This malalignment issue is primarily a result of our facial jaw bones shrinking over the past few centuries. My esteemed colleagues Dr. Kevin Boyd and Dr. Marianna Evans have dedicated their research on comparing our faces with our fairly recent (200- to 300-year-old) forefathers—who had no need for orthodontics. We covered this at length in the chapter on Breathe, but this begs a recap on *why* it happened.

Anthropological evidence now points to processed food and a lack of breastfeeding as the culprit. Generations of children were weaned from a bottle and pacifier (with less reliance on breastfeeding) and fed blended, pureed "baby" food. Without sucking from a breast and chewing fibrous foods, our tongue and jaw muscles are not developing to their potential and are reducing the size of our children's faces, tongue boxes, and yes, dental arches.

Dental crowding became an obvious consequence. Keeping in mind that small jaw bones are also intimately connected to the soft tissues of the upper airway complex: nose, sinuses, back of the throat, etc. Dr. Boyd has termed this the craniofacial-respiratory complex, or CFRC. In addition to crooked teeth, shrinking of the CFRC has created an avalanche of breathing problems, sleep-related breathing disorders, and obstructive sleep apnea, which you can review in more detail in the Breathe and Sleep chapters.

The contemporary concept of braces ranges from metal bands, brackets, and wires to the increasingly popular "invisible" clear aligners. White braces and lingual (tongue-side) braces are alternative aesthetic options. Ortho is treatment primarily focused on these kiddos who have dental crowding and unsatisfactory jawbone growth. It's not considered difficult to align front teeth for a pretty smile display. But maximizing the airway and reengineering a stable occlusion (bite relationship) are two entirely more challenging concepts. The best orthodontists are working harder than ever to solve these complexities.

Years after orthodontics, many people find their teeth crowding again and ask me for help. I find they usually blame themselves for disregarding their retainers—as if they should be reliant on a little piece of plastic for the rest of their adult life. But that's not the primary cause. Dental professions agree that good orthodontic outcomes with balanced opposing bite forces are much better predictors of long-term stability than any style of orthodontic retainer.

Ideal orthodontic outcomes mean:

- balanced facial bones

- a well-fitting, balanced bite
- teeth surrounded by an adequate housing of bone
- an aesthetically pleasing amount of tooth and gum "display" in speaking and smiling
- a broad palate that's adequately shaped for the tongue to be resting up against
- a broad, toothy smile with no dark corridors near the corners of the mouth
- jaw dimensions that allow lips to close easily at rest
- and last, but not least, straight alignment of teeth

That's a tall order!

To achieve all this, progressive orthodontists are diving into a deeper initial evaluation that involves an airway assessment, soft tissue support (including tongue function, tongue-ties, resting tongue posture, tonsils, adenoids, and facial soft tissue), and the entire complex of bones that support the face—not just the teeth.

Meanwhile, most Brave Parents would choose not to have our children wear braces if we could have a beautiful smile, balanced bite, and open airway without them. I'm compelled to reiterate that we now believe the majority of dental malalignment is indeed *preventable*, if we are paying attention to breathing, sleeping, chewing, and swallowing patterns from babyhood—and intervening at younger ages as needed.

To avoid braces, toddlers and school-age children can engage in myofunctional therapy, early expansion of the upper jaw, mouth taping, successful release of tongue-ties, and removal of engorged tonsils and adenoids. Catch all of this and more in the Breathe chapter if you haven't yet done so.

Meanwhile, bravest of all Brave Parents, choosing airway-educated health professionals, including your orthodontist, makes good sense—even if it means driving past many other orthodontists on your way to and from appointments.

66

Meanwhile, most **Brave Parents** would **choose not to have** our children wear **braces** if we could have a beautiful **smile**, balanced **bite**, and open **airway** without them. I'm compelled to reiterate that we now believe the majority of dental malalignment is indeed *preventable,* if we are paying attention to **breathing, sleeping, chewing, and swallowing** patterns from babyhood—and intervening at younger ages as needed.

99

7.19 PREVENTING OROPHARYNGEAL CANCER (OPC) FOR YOUR CHILD'S FUTURE

Human papillomavirus (HPV) is our most common sexually transmitted infection (STI), affecting over seventy-nine million Americans. As a result, the incidence of all HPV-related cancers (such as cervical, anal, penile, vaginal, and oropharyngeal) has escalated at an alarming rate over the last four decades.

The US CDC states that HPV infection is now so common that nearly all US men and women will get at least one type of HPV at some point in their lives.

Sadly, the rate of sexually transmitted infections among adolescents is also increasing at an unprecedented rate, including this one. According to US CDC there are over six million new cases of HPV infections each year, and it's estimated that 74% of them occur in fifteen- to twenty-four-year-olds.

Mimicking that infection trend, the incidence of resulting oropharyngeal cancer is soaring at an increase of 30% a year. In 2011 medical scientists predicted HPV-OPC would surpass HPV-cervical cancers by 2020! The prediction was wrong. Oral pharyngeal cancers surpassed cervical cancers five years *earlier,* in 2015, and is now the most common HPV-malignancy in the US. Whereas cervical cancer was a woman's risk, 82% of these oropharyngeal cancers occur in men.

So, what's this grouping of viruses all about? Scientists have identified over 200 strains of HPV, and they live on your skin and mine. If you put a piece of masking tape anywhere on your body and picked it up, you'd undoubtably find it lurking there. (Hmm, there's that masking tape again! LOL)

Some of these strains invade the skin to cause warts on your child's fingers or feet. But a handful of these strains (especially HPV-16 and HPV-18) are not so harmless—they are highly cancer-causing. They flourish on wet, bumpy surfaces, like that covering a cervix or *oropharynx* (the back of the throat, base of the tongue, or around the tonsils). A viral cluster can hang around for years and then either clear up on their own (like warts sometimes do) or morph the surrounding cells into a devastating cancer.

I was lucky enough to practice for thirty years without diagnosing a single oral cancer. But in the last six years, I've averaged one per year. The radiation treatment for head and neck cancer alone will bring a person to their knees! Even after that, two of my dear friends (patients) did not survive the cancer.

Because you're an adult, your dental hygienist routinely scans your mouth for oral cancer. This practice began some fifty years ago, stemming from the days when oral cancer was primarily caused by tobacco and alcohol. Today only 30% of the oral cancers appear in the mouth itself. The other 70% are these HPV-cancer lesions, literally *hidden* in the base of the tongue or back of the throat. Sadly, there are no effective screening methods or tests for detecting those cancers until they advance to cause signs or symptoms.

In our total health dental practice, I'm able to assay your saliva for possible *infection* of the cancer-causing HPV strains. But that will only alert you to become hyperaware of developing signs or symptoms, such as enlarged neck nodes. Unfortunately, it's not like a Pap smear, where the surface of the cervix is scraped to detect early cancer cells.

So, our best defense against HPV-OPC is *education* and *vaccination*. First let's talk about education.

7.20 SEX EDUCATION AT HOME

If my mom were still alive, her couples-counselor-and-sex-therapist self would have insisted I give this book an entire chapter on Sexual Health. I am choosing to dodge that topic, not because it's unimportant, but because I am afraid to offend some of you and thereby discredit the entire book in your eyes.

But on this subject, I feel zealous in my urging you to BE BRAVE and talk about sex. Open the dialogue about differences between males and females when your child is young, and answer questions one at a time as your child becomes curious. Don't be surprised if their curiosities around some delicate subjects surface far earlier than you want them to—it happens for all parents.

Your goal will be to sustain an *ongoing dialogue*–one where your kiddo feels *safe* asking YOU (instead of their peers) and *confident* that you will answer truthfully. You might start with a sincere "Thank you for asking me." Then, answer their sex questions matter-of-factly, trying your best not to laugh or to shame your kiddo for the inquiry. Also, try not to give a bunch more detail than he or she is asking. You don't want to freak them out. My mom over-answered a few times, and it felt like a shocker.

When it was my turn to parent, I tried to give my son straight answers to his every inquiry. Here's a funny example from the mouth of my eight-year-old Hunter:

"Okay Mom, level with me! I want to know the *whole* story about how babies are made, and here's what I know so far: The man has the seed, and the woman has the egg. And the seed has to *get* to the egg to grow the baby, I get that. Oh ... and I also know they have to be lying in front of the fire ... and the fire has to be *burning*." (Hilarious? It was hard not to laugh at that, and I still have no idea where that came from.)

Then he continued, "But *how* does the man's seed actually get to the woman's egg? Does he just lie next to her and pee on her, or what?" He was clearly asking for the rest of the story.

You might notice your kiddo's questions start to dwindle in middle school when they start to talk (or text) with their close friends instead of you. Then I would encourage you to assume they still have questions and initiate the conversation.

Doing our best to maintain an open dialogue will erase the awkwardness when it's time for you to give your growing-up child healthful advice along the way. Messages like, "Oral sex isn't safe sex!" And now we're back on the subject of HPV oropharyngeal cancer risks.

" In today's culture there is an ever-growing *acceptance* of **"body part sex,"** given that about **14% of thirteen-year-olds**, and **41% of fifteen-year-olds** have already participated. "

In today's culture there is an ever-growing acceptance of "body part sex," given that about 14% of thirteen-year-olds, and 41% of fifteen-year-olds have already participated.

We are amidst a cultural shift toward oral sex being considered safe and casual, even amongst middle schoolers of *every* demographic.

You might not want to hear this, but many twelve- and thirteen-year-old girls now consider fellatio the necessary price of hanging on to a cool boyfriend or appearing more mature to her friends. Oral sex also seems to quell some of the pressure to "go all the way."

Boys need straight talk, too, since they engage in oral sex at about the same or at even slightly higher rates. Historically, STIs were more prevalent in women, but today, HPV-OPC favors middle-aged men, many of whom were infected as teens.

The reason for this is indeed being pinned on sexual behavior. It's stated in the literature that "white men have the highest number of lifetime oral sex partners and first report performing oral sex at a younger age, compared with other racial/ethnic groups."

7.21 HPV VACCINATION IS KEY

In 2006 our US FDA approved the first Gardasil vaccine, targeting eleven- and twelve-year-old girls and boys for the two-shot vaccination series.

The HPV vaccine campaign focused primarily on the prevention of cervical cancer in women, even though the FDA allowed the vaccine indications to include prevention of HPV cancers of the vulva, vagina, penis, and anus.

Progressive pediatricians and family docs spread the word about cervical cancer prevention. They stressed vaccination for girls more than boys—since boys were viewed as potential HPV *carriers*, not the targets. There was even inequity in the CDC's vaccine recommendation (and subsequent reimbursement), covering boys up to age eighteen and girls to twenty-six.

Also frustrating was the stance by more conservative docs, that the vaccine would actually *promote* early sexual behavior among children. (As if kids really know what each of their shots are for.)

While I'm on a rant, this bugged me to no end: HPV oropharyngeal cancer (OPC) was left completely off the list of cancers this vaccine could prevent, so the media never talked about it. Scientists *knew* oropharyngeal cancer was sexually transmitted and caused by the exact same high-risk HPV strains covered by the vaccine, but the FDA kept calling for more studies related specifically to the cancers of the oropharynx before they would include it.

Alas, in late 2020, the agency *finally* approved the vaccine for protection from HPV-OPC. That means we will *finally* hear the media and advertisements recommending the vaccine for prevention from these brutal, often late-detected throat cancers.

We also made prevention headway when, in 2016, the FDA upped the age recommended for the Gardasil 9 vaccine to forty-five.

If it sounds like I'm a fan of this particular vaccine, I am. I'm sick of cancer! And fortunately, the 9-valent HPV vaccine targets the *oncogenic* (cancer-causing) types attributed to 74% of the HPV-associated cancers we see today.

You don't need to visit your physician for the Gardasil 9 series, as any pharmacies that administer vaccines can help. If you were vaccinated prior to October 2018, you received Gardasil 4, meaning *four* HPV strains, but you may want to consult your physician or pharmacist about a booster, as the Gardasil 9 includes five more high-risk strains.

CONCLUSION

It's hard to reign myself in on the variety of topics that have become my life's work. I hope you feel my passion for oral health—a space that has sorely been pushed aside by virtually all of medicine. Knowing the tremendous impact oral disease has on our bodies, it's high time we bridge the gaps between dentistry and medicine. If you're interested in learning much more about mouth-body connections, please read my first book, *BlabberMouth! 77 Secrets Only Your Mouth Can Tell You to Live a Healthier, Happier, Sexier Life.*

66

Sadly, the rate of **sexually transmitted infections** among adolescents is also

increasing

at an unprecedented rate, including this one. According to US CDC there are over **six million new cases of HPV** infections each year, and it's estimated that

74%

of them occur in **fifteen- to twenty-four**-year-olds.

99

CHAPTER 7 REFERENCES

AAPD. (2021). *Perinatal and Infant Oral Health Care - AAPD.* Perinatal and Infant Oral Health Care. Retrieved November 4, 2021, from https://www.aapd.org/globalassets/media/policies_guidelines/bp_perinataloralhealthcare.pdf.

Azarpazhooh, A., & Main, P. A. (2009). Efficacy of dental prophylaxis (Rubber Cup) for the prevention of caries and gingivitis: A systematic review of literature. *British Dental Journal, 207*(7). https://doi.org/10.1038/sj.bdj.2009.899.

Bale, B. F., Doneen, A. L., & Vigerust, D. J. (2016). High-risk periodontal pathogens contribute to the pathogenesis of Atherosclerosis. *Postgraduate Medical Journal, 93*(1098), 215–220. https://doi.org/10.1136/postgradmedj-2016-134279.

CDC. (2019, September 10). *Dental Caries in Primary Teeth.* Centers for Disease Control and Prevention. Retrieved October 15, 2021, from https://www.cdc.gov/oralhealth/publications/OHSR-2019-summary.html.

CDC. (2021, April 5). *HPV statistics.* Centers for Disease Control and Prevention. Retrieved November 3, 2021, from https://www.cdc.gov/std/hpv/stats.htm.

CDC. (2021, October 1). *Water fluoridation basics.* Centers for Disease Control and Prevention. Retrieved November 15, 2021, from https://www.cdc.gov/fluoridation/basics/index.htm.

Center for Biologics Evaluation and Research. (2009, August 20). *Gardasil Vaccine Safety.* U.S. Food and Drug Administration. Retrieved November 1, 2021, from https://www.fda.gov/vaccines-blood-biologics/safety-availability-biologics/gardasil-vaccine-safety.

Clark, M. B., & Slayton, R. L. (2014). Fluoride use in caries prevention in the Primary Care Setting. *PEDIATRICS, 134*(3), 626–633. https://doi.org/10.1542/peds.2014-1699.

Dye, B. A. (2017). The global burden of oral disease: Research and public health significance. *Journal of Dental Research, 96*(4), 361–363. https://doi.org/10.1177/0022034517693567.

Horowitz, H. S. (1996). The effectiveness of community water fluoridation in the United States. *Journal of Public Health Dentistry, 56*(5), 253–258. https://doi.org/10.1111/j.1752-7325.1996.tb02448.x.

Jeevarathan, J., Deepti, A., Muthu, M. S., Prabhu, V. R., & Chamundeeswari, G. S. (2007). Effect of fluoride varnish on streptococcus mutans counts in plaque of caries-free children using dentocult SM strip mutans test: A randomized controlled triple blind study. *Journal of Indian Society of Pedodontics and Preventive Dentistry, 25*(4), 157. https://doi.org/10.4103/0970-4388.37010.

Kutsch, K. V. (2020). *Why Me? The unfair reason you get cavities and what to do about it.* WellPut Custom Content.

Lamster, I. B., Lalla, E., Borgnakke, W. S., & Taylor, G. W. (2008). The relationship between Oral Health and diabetes mellitus. *The Journal of the American Dental Association, 139.* https://doi.org/10. 14219/jada.archive.2008.0363.

Mansour-Ghanaei, F., Joukar, F., Atshani, S. M., Chagharvand, S., & Souti, F. (2013, September 12). *The epidemiology of gastroesophageal reflux disease: A survey on the prevalence and the associated factors in a random sample of the general population in the northern part of Iran.* International journal of molecular epidemiology and genetics. Retrieved November 15, 2021, from https://www.ncbi.nlm.nih.gov/pmc/articles/PMC3773569/.

Maples, S. S., & DeCouteau, D. K. (2015). *BlabberMouth!: 77 Secrets Only Your Mouth Can Tell You To Live a Healthier, Happier, Sexier Life.* Blabbermouth.

National Institute of Dental and Craniofacial research. (2018). *The story of fluoridation.* National Institute of Dental and Craniofacial Research. Retrieved October 15, 2021, from https://www.nidcr.nih.gov/health-info/fluoride/the-story-of-fluoridation.

Price, W. A. (1939). *Nutrition and physical degeneration: A comparison of primitive and modern diet and their effects.* s.n.

Schuster, M. A., Bell, R. M., & Kanouse, D. E. (1996). The sexual practices of adolescent virgins: Genital sexual activities of high school students who have never had vaginal intercourse. *American*

Journal of Public Health, 86(11), 1570–1576. https://doi.org/10.2105/ajph.86.11.1570.

U.S. Department of Health and Human Services. *Oral Health in America: A Report of the Surgeon General.* Rockville, MD: U.S. Department of Health and Human Services, National Institute of Dental and Craniofacial Research, National Institutes of Health, 2000. https://www.nidcr.nih.gov/research/data-statistics/surgeon-general.

Van Dyne, E. A., Henley, S. J., Saraiya, M., Thomas, C. C., Markowitz, L. E., & Benard, V. B. (2018). Trends in human papillomavirus–associated cancers — United States, 1999–2015. *MMWR. Morbidity and Mortality Weekly Report, 67*(33), 918–924. https://doi.org/10.15585/mmwr.mm6733a2.

Varadan, M., & Ramamurthy, J. (2014). Association of periodontal disease and pre-term low birth weight infants. *The Journal of Obstetrics and Gynecology of India, 65*(3), 167–171. https://doi.org/10.1007/s13224-014-0581-9.

Vergnes, J.-N., & Mazevet, M. (2020). Oral diseases: A global public health challenge. *The Lancet, 395*(10219), 186. https://doi.org/10.1016/s0140-6736(19)33015-6.

Wilkerson, D. W. C., & Lestini, S. E. (2019). *The shift: The dramatic movement toward health centered dentistry.* St. Petersburg, Fla.

Zokaie, T., & Pollick, H. (2021). Community water fluoridation and the integrity of Equitable Public Health Infrastructure. *Journal of Public Health Dentistry.* https://doi.org/10.1111/jphd.12480.

CHAPTER EIGHT

move

FOSTERING A DAILY DOSE OF GET-UP-N-GO!

INTRODUCTION

I've saved this chapter for the last. Not because it's the least important or the last thing you should champion in your Brave Parent journey to your child's optimal health. But last because it's a precious subject to me.

Exercise saved my life!

Of the people who are born with chronic health complications that could easily have killed them in childhood, few are fortunate enough to overcome those obstacles. And even fewer people are blessed enough to meet a stranger who becomes their *surrogate Brave Parent* just when they are needed the most. If you remember from this book's introduction, this is *my* story. And by coaching me to achieve her prescription of thirty minutes of strenuous activity a day, my chronic diseases slowly began to wane ... and a few years later, they vanished altogether.

In these last few pages, I need to convince you that your child deserves that, too, even if they weren't born with a chronic condition or a surrogate Brave Parent. They have YOU. And you're plenty!

> 66 We need **aerobic** activity and **muscle-building** activity in equal measures. And we need at least one of them each and **every day.** As a human cohort, we are wired for **movement**, not to be molded into a couch or a chair. Staying on the couch might feel good for the moment, but every time you force yourself to get up and get going,
>
> *you won't regret it.*
>
> "Gosh, I wish I hadn't worked out," said no one... *ever.* 99

If you're a wannabe daily exerciser, and you're now feeling guilty for not making that happen for yourself, you're in good company. According to Alex Azar, Secretary of the US Department of Health and Human Services, 80% of adults are not meeting the key guidelines for *both* aerobic and muscle-strengthening activity, and only about half meet the guidelines for aerobic activity.

Chances are you didn't grow up with a habit of daily exercise that weaved its way into your adulthood. I'm sure it feels hard to start now amidst *all* your other responsibilities. But NOW might be the perfect time to start!

This is not intended to add any more not-enoughness to your conscience. But the best way to stop "shoulding" on yourself is to close this book and go walk (or ride or dance) for *ten* minutes. Every ten minutes makes a difference!

Daily movement is a perfect way to become a healthier, happier person ... and a brave example to your kiddos. It also says, "I'm serious about this lifestyle enhancement for us! Because I don't want either of us to become a lifestyle-disease statistic. Wait ... No! It's not about statistics; it's because I want the *very best quality of life for you.*"

With *half* our population overweight, we have processed food and drinks to accuse. But we also have our sedentary, convenient, couch-sitting, screen-addicted habits sharing the helm.

We need aerobic activity *and* muscle-building activity in equal measures. And we need at least one of them *each and every day.* As a human cohort, we are wired for movement, not to be molded into a couch or a chair. Staying on the couch might feel good for the moment, but every time you force yourself to get up and get going, you won't regret it. "Gosh, I wish I hadn't worked out," said no one ... ever!

> 66 While **handheld electronics** make a *captivating babysitter*, it's clearly not how these littles are supposed to live. It's such a dilemma. I get that the ability to **"sedate" a child into stillness** is incredibly tempting, but when the screen becomes a **regular companion,** a child sort of **forgets** how they're supposed **to be.** 99

Habitual exercise is a critical weapon in combatting the childhood obesity crisis we see today, but believe me, it's a critical component of health, even if your kiddo is underweight! Our bodies are designed with engines that need revving. And the more our engines sit idle, the more our metabolic, emotional, and cognitive health weakens.

In 2010, First Lady Michelle Obama launched the *Let's Move!* Campaign, and President Barack Obama established the Task Force on Childhood Obesity. Their unbelievably ambitious goal was to solve the problem of childhood obesity *within one generation*. Once again, awareness was not enough to turn the trends. And you can bet their daring attempts at public policy reform were met with resistance from the food, beverage, and sugar lobbyists galore.

What *will* be enough to upend the trend? That has yet to be answered. I'm thinking it will be through a fervent grassroots effort. Maybe you and I can help ... by engaging in an entire Brave Parent movement.

Let these dire statistics sink in. In 2016, there were over 340 million US children and adolescents overweight or obese (85th percentile and above). If that's not enough to make you cry, thirty-nine million children—under the age of five—are counted in the overweight or obese population. I hate to say it, but almost every single one of *these* littles are doomed from the start.

And oh, by the way, we have yet to determine the COVID-effect on childhood obesity, but it doesn't appear to be good.

Today is August 12, 2021, and my kiddos (patients) are scheduled to start in-person school next week. Most of them have endured a full COVID-year of at-home virtual learning. So, I asked one of my fourth-grade patients yesterday if he was excited go back to school, face-to-face. He responded with a placid shrug of indifference, "I guess so. But I'm not gonna lie. It was really nice to just wake up, grab my laptop, and go to school all day from my own bed."

His answer, along with his overtones of depression, continues to haunt me. As a sign of the times, it is disturbing on so many levels. I hate to play the "back when I was a child ..." card, but right now I can't help it. Back when I was a child, the steepest punishment we would receive was, "Go to your room!" Now it's hard to get kids to come out of their rooms. In fact, (and now *I'm* not gonna lie) that little guy sounded a lot like my elderly patients in palliative care who are just trying to stay comfortable in their last days of life.

Again, when is this horrific trend going to stop? And do you want to help? It's crazy to me that we now have federally published *physical activity guidelines* for our children ... even our *toddlers*, ages one to three. Wow! (But I get it.)

In my dental office, I regularly see toddlers sitting stunned, like silent statues, while they wait. It's not because of their lessons in good manners or their self-discipline. It's because their attention is laser-focused on an electronic tablet, playing a game or movie.

While handheld electronics make a captivating babysitter, it's clearly *not* how these littles are supposed to live. It's such a dilemma. I get that the ability to "sedate" a child into stillness is incredibly tempting, but when the screen becomes a regular companion, a child sort of forgets how they're supposed to be.

I have come to know this with everything that I am. My own toddler life wasn't healthy either. It was screwed up with sleep deprivation, prescription medications, doctor visits, and trying to avoid outdoor allergens. I was often out of gas. I, too, became sedentary and overweight (by yesteryear's standards). Ultimately, I had to remember my essence ... which is to move.

In this chapter, let me describe to you, from a very personal and very passionate place, just what daily physical activity promises to give your children. And you.

Daily exercise bestows such incredible physical, emotional, and spiritual gifts!

With our goal to foster in your children a lifetime habit of daily exercise, I want to help you discover what your kiddo can (and should) be embracing in their early years in order to make it happen.

> **" Daily exercise** bestows such incredible physical, emotional, and spiritual *gifts!* **"**

8.1 A STORY ABOUT A DOG

Oh good, you're still reading. I thought if I labeled this "The Benefits of Physical Activity," you'd roll your eyes and skip this section altogether. Aren't you sick of the academic bullet points about what you can gain from regular exercise? I am. It's a scrolling list with no more big surprises.

So, I'll boil down the research and tell you succinctly: kids who exercise develop *all* elements of metabolic health—better heart and lung fitness, stronger bones, more restful sleep, emotional stability, *and* improved cognitive function. Engrave this summary into your Brave Parent memory bank because ... it's all true! If my dog could speak English, she'd tell you too.

As I write this, I'm enjoying watching this effervescent fifteen-year-old "puppy" literally prance around the deck, jumping on and off, chasing critters. (Ellie also naps a lot—fair game since she's over eighty in human years.) Her only veterinary visits have been for annual well-visits, vaccinations, and teeth cleaning. She weighs nine pounds—one-half pound more than she weighed at her first birthday.

Ellie's doc attributes her longevity, frolicking energy, and good health to my determination to give her forty-five minutes (minimum) of exercise a day. That was easy as a baby and even through her "teenage" years (about two to three). And by then the habit was ingrained. She kept running with me, four to five miles a day, through her adulthood too. This fall, for her sixteenth birthday gift, I'm restoring her eyesight with cataract surgery so she can feel even younger next year.

I'm telling you Ellie's story because I truly believe *all* members of the animal kingdom, including you and me, thrive with movement … and fail without it.

I bet you're sick of me droning on about our out-of-control rates of lifestyle-related killer diseases. But guess who *doesn't* have *any* of these? The countless wild animals who roam the planet unfettered.

Why? Because they have to *move* all day just to get food. They have no choice. They have no convenience stores.

And because every bite they eat is right from the source. Talk about *whole foods*! There is no added sugar, and nothing in their diet is processed.

By the way, this phenomenon doesn't hold true for the pets we keep in captivity, our dogs and cats. They sit on the couch right next to us and eat the commercial pet food we buy from the grocery store. In case you thought they'd been spared in the obesity crisis, the 2016 State of Pet Health Report indicated an upward trend in diabetes prevalence, rising almost 80% in dogs and 18% in cats over a ten-year period. Pets who avoid obesity and diabetes get plenty of exercise and avoid carbed-up food. (I apologize if you're suddenly experiencing added pressure to become a Brave Pet Parent too.)

> **66** Today, about half of us—**117 million people**—have one or more preventable *chronic diseases*. And get this: seven of the ten of these most common chronic diseases are **positively impacted** by **regular exercise**. **99**

Back to people. Today, about *half* of us—117 million people— have one or more *preventable* chronic diseases. And get this: seven of the ten of these most common chronic diseases are positively impacted by regular exercise.

If dollars and cents is a motivator, consider that our sedentary lifestyle is costing us a fortune. Our lack of physical activity (by itself) is to blame for about $117 *billion* in annual health care costs.

What does that $117 billion buy? Heart bypass surgery, limb amputation from uncontrolled diabetes, bariatric surgery for obesity, knee and hip replacements from obesity, blindness from diabetic retinopathy, and a plethora of medications for hypertension, high cholesterol, and depression. And the list goes on and on and on.

Let's get to work to figure out how to avoid *all* of this for your children, for you, and even for your pets.

8.2 A STORY ABOUT A MAN AND HIS DOG

Hey, if it worked once, it's bound to work again. LOL. Here's a doggie tale about how regular activity helps reduce (or prevent) insulin resistance, type 2 diabetes, and fat storage.

For most adults who exercise sporadically, their motivation is to look better. They often grow impatient waiting for the results of their hard work to show up on their bodies. It seems to take forever!

In contrast, changes in blood chemistry are *instantaneous*, even during short stints of moderate activity. For example, if you take a walk after a primary meal, your working muscles will gobble up your circulating blood sugar, making it less likely you'll convert that sugar to stored fat. That also means you won't overtax your body's insulin-glucose-feedback loop that, when off-kilter, marches you right toward *insulin resistance.*

So, when we enforce daily activity for ourselves and our kids, we're truly attending to our *internal health* even more than our *external appeal.*

One of my adult patients came to his six-month preventive appointment proud as a peacock over his thirty-pound weight loss. I was excited to hear his story, so I asked, as I always do, "How'd you do it?"

He quipped back, "Wait ... you don't remember? It was *your* prescription, Doc."

"Prescription?" I asked, even more confused. "I only remember we tested your A1c (a two- to three-month average of circulating blood sugar) and found you were in the pre-diabetic range."

"Yep," he continued, "and *then* you told me I could drop that number if I was willing to take just two brisk, ten-minute walks a day. To which I replied, 'I hate to walk.' And then *you* said, 'Well, then just get a dog. You know, people don't walk dogs ... *dogs walk people!*'"

"As soon as I got home, I told my wife that my dentist prescribed a puppy! She was over-the-moon excited because she'd been wanting one, and voila ... three weeks later we had our new best friend. Now, my puppy walks me five times a day. I've already lost thirty pounds, and my hygienist, Sara, just gave me the stellar news about my A1c. Will you just look at that!"

It's a fun story that you can share with your family too. And if you and your kids have pets, resist the urge to take all responsibility. Kids who care for their pets develop character, practice account-ability for another vulnerable being, learn more about love, *and* reap profound health benefits. (See chapter Digest for more health perks gained by living with a dog.)

8.3 WHAT KIND OF EXERCISE DOES YOUR KIDDO NEED?

First, the *daily* kind. Forget about three days a week. We're going for everyday exercise ... for the rest of their ever-loving lives. Just as you wouldn't think of letting your kiddo go without food, water, or sleep in any given day, please start to think about daily exercise as essential for your child's overall well-being.

I'm not alone in my recommendation. The US CDC Youth Physical Activity Guidelines suggest that children and adolescents ages six through seventeen should have a *minimum* of one hour of moderate-to-vigorous intensity physical activity *each day*.

That's for your kiddos' health TODAY. But it's an enormous investment in their future health, too, since we've learned that children who exercise regularly are significantly more likely to seek physical activity and fitness throughout their life span.

The past forty years of exercise physiology research have made two concepts emerge with crystal clarity: (1) every bit of exercise is helpful, even in snippets of ten-minute increments and (2) more is always better.

Don't be afraid to assert your expectations for daily exercise and hold kids accountable. In my "field research" for this chapter, I queried all the committed everyday-exercisers I know about how they came to their ongoing physical fitness.

I started with my son, who simply answered. "Is that a serious question, Mom? I sort of had no choice. Between you and Dad, exercise was elevated to bible status in our family."

I like that he knew what was expected. And believe me, we weren't running a hard labor camp—we always tried to make it fun first and challenging second.

"*Children* who **exercise regularly** are significantly more likely to **seek physical activity** and fitness **throughout their** *life span*."

If your kiddos aren't babies anymore and you're getting a late start on these expectations, sit down together and carve out a plan. And by all means count yourself in!

Don't be surprised if you experience some pushback. If you find your children are glued to the screen or more engrossed in exercising their thumbs than exercising their bodies (tapping out messages on a handheld), consider negotiating for an *equal* measure of screen time with exercise time.

8.4 CARDIO VERSUS STRENGTH TRAINING

Your kiddo needs *both* cardio (or endurance) training and weight (or strength) training.

Cardio doesn't mean your kiddo has to be breathless and red-faced, but they should increase their respiration and heart rates above resting. This can be achieved by any activity that includes running, swimming, cycling, energized walking, boxing, dancing, skating, or jumping rope.

Cardio is *aerobic* exercise. It fortifies the cardiovascular system by expanding the lungs, gobbling up circulating blood sugar, and strengthening the heart muscle. It also bolsters your mood, sleep, joints, and bone health.

Aerobic activity burns calories and lowers blood sugar in the moment without necessarily building muscle. Starting your day with a challenging cardio workout also revs your engine early, boosting your oxygen circulation and allowing you to burn calories at a higher rate throughout the day.

In contrast, *strength training* means weight-bearing activity. In whatever way you choose to stress the restrictions of your muscles, you will stimulate repair. If you really overdo it, your muscles will scream at you tomorrow. But if you're cool about it, you'll be ever-so-slightly sore, somewhere in your body, every day. And, my dear ones, this is how skeletal muscles grow. As an added bonus, your emerging muscles will pull on your bones, stimulating bone growth too.

The benefits of strength training for kids are numerous. It bolsters coordination, motor control, mental health, bone health, balance, reduced risk of injuries, and self-esteem. There's one more colossal benefit, and it's critically important in today's world: It lowers fat mass.

How does that work? Muscle cells burn three and a half times more calories—at rest—than fat. Think about that for a minute. If you and I are both reading a book right now, we are both sitting relatively idle. Whichever one of us has *more* muscle mass is burning more calories during our reading session, and thus able to enjoy more calories from foods without depositing body fat. We've simply built a bigger engine that requires more fuel, even at rest.

So, if you want to avoid "portion control" (such an unappealing concept) without gaining fat, put on some more muscle. For every pound of added muscle, you will burn about ten extra calories a day. Gain ten pounds of muscle and burn about one hundred extra calories at rest.

When we think of strength training these days, our minds conjure up images of repeated gym workouts with barbells, racks, and dumbbells. Even if you have a home gym, that's probably not the place for your little kiddos.

There have been some evidence-based concerns that weight lifting is not good for children before they enter puberty. Even then, they need instruction and monitoring. Studies have suggested that early weight training might interrupt a child's growth or lead to injuries.

But kids can certainly start with bodyweight exercises, such as sit-ups, push-ups, squats, burpees, wall sits, stair walking, and triceps dips. They can also engage in the practice of yoga. Beyond bodyweight strength training, the growing body of research has already shown that yoga can improve focus, memory, self-esteem, academic performance, classroom behavior, and can even reduce anxiety and stress in children.

66

The benefits of strength training for kids are *numerous.*

It bolsters **coordination, motor control, mental health, bone health, balance, reduced risk of injuries**, and **self-esteem**. There's one more colossal benefit, and it's **critically important** in today's world:

It **lowers** *FAT MASS.*

99

I'm a big fan of light resistance bands, too, especially for upper body strength training during an outdoor walk. That's a fun all-encompassing, upper-body-lower-body aerobic activity you can do as a family. Yes, you'll look peculiar to your neighbors, in such a bold, Brave Parent way! You can rock that!

If you are curious about the latest research on all these concepts, read *Which Comes First, Cardio or Weights?* by Alex Hutchinson. It's not about children, but it'll give you a fantastic foundational understanding of exercise physiology.

8.5 ORGANIZED SPORTS

I have developed a love-hate relationship with organized sports.

I just love the character-building opportunities that come from being part of a team: responsibility to others, what it means to become a team player, how to follow rules, how to lose gracefully and win humbly, how to respectfully receive coaching, and SO much more.

Exceptional coaches can become surrogate Brave Parents also. You might know this from experience.

My nephew Michael asked me to remind you that *helicopter parents* (those who hover) often don't allow enough room for other awesome adults to have a profound influence on their child. In today's world, coaches (and teachers) are more reluctant to impart their philosophies to kids for fear they might be politically incorrect or, in some other way, rub parents the wrong way. If your kiddo gets a lucky draw on an athletic coach (or band director, teacher, etc.) you feel particularly grateful for, thank them, and give them permission to teach integrity, sportsmanship, humility, and any other positive expressions of conduct.

I also really like the self-esteem building that results from continual hard work and a sense of personal contribution to a competitive team. Forget the proverbial "trophy for every participant." *This* is the real prize!

Being part of a winning team begs *courage, spirit,* and *grit* from each individual, and these are super important attributes for a child to develop. (Of course, that notion is not exclusive to team success or even physical activity. *Anything* tough we set out to accomplish in life, and then do so, reinforces self-esteem, courage, spirit, and grit.)

Now on to the *hate* relationship with our cultural emphasis on team sports. Perhaps what I loathe most is the dominance that professional sports have taken over the spirit of true recreation and kind-practice socialization in today's world. In that vein, we've somehow elevated our pro athletes to godlike status symbols—even when their appalling public behaviors serve as worst-case examples to our all-eyes-on-them children. I could cite countless examples, but then, so could you. You know what I'm talking about.

I also dislike how our enchantment with pro sports has diminished our enthusiasm for the arts: music, theater, dance, painting, sculpture, creative writing, and the like.

I've noticed that many families who have a dedicated emphasis on sports performance hold professional sports viewing as a central theme for their family entertainment. The pro-sports arena has become a contemporary culture unto itself—and one that doesn't exactly subscribe to the Scouts' honor code. I'm troubled by the mind-blowing amount of money that exchanges hands in thousands of icky ways, legally and illegally, over "professional" games. If you're engaged in pro sports as a family, be sure to point out breaches in integrity as you see them and express your disappointment.

As well, teach your kids not to judge others based on their team affiliations. This should go without saying ... but it doesn't. As much as I enjoy respectful team rivalry, I'm disheartened that we're each somewhat pressured into identifying with specific teams we "belong" to, while we garner abject disdain from others for just being labeled as a fan of team X. It seems like no matter where I go, I'm asked if I'm a "Michigan fan." (I suppose that's because my audience members know it's my dental school alma mater.) Then, depending on my answer, I'm addressed with more respect ... or less.

While cultivating team spirit can be fun, it's important you teach that this kind of judgment is not only *exclusive* but unnecessary and meaningless since our affiliation with a sports team says *nothing* about us as people, right!?

Finally, I'm really opposed to adults encouraging talented school-age athletes to think about a career as a professional athlete. (I've noticed that parents often report their kid's aspiration as a badge of honor.) The fame and fortune of their favorite MVPs can become entirely alluring for some young athletes. A career in athletics is a pipe dream, and if they sway heavily toward athletics and against education, it can become a devastating one at that. You, Brave Parent, need to brace your child for the truth.

Only one in 16,000 high school athletes ever makes it to the pros. And while it's awesome that elite sports performance can earn talented players a college scholarship, the fact is only two in one hundred athletes even go on to play a college sport of any kind, at any level. Contrast that with the 59% of high school football and basketball players who truly believe they'll earn a full-ride college scholarship.

I am not suggesting that you become a killjoy to your kiddo's pro-sports fantasy, but it's up to you to help them keep one foot grounded in reality. You, Brave Parent, need to be the voice of reason, encouraging their athletic prowess *while* you cheerlead for their education—reading, writing, math, and reasoning skills. And while you're at it, encourage them to explore their interests in the arts too. These provide other ways to express passion, perseverance, performance, and creativity.

All this considered, I absolutely supported my son's desire to play year-round organized sports of several varieties. Because it was *his* desire, not his dad's or mine. He was a competitive kid who had a strong work ethic, and he didn't let his academics suffer for his sports.

Okay, please welcome me back to my love for organized sports. A handful of my field research team (interviewed about how they came to exercise daily), gave credit to an awesome sports team experience. A few said they responded to the physical challenges posed by great coaches. And more significantly, some really loved the way "being in great shape" *felt* to them, and they never wanted to lose that feeling.

My advice is to surround your child's sports practices and competitions with *individualized* outside physical activity that *supports* their success—and preferably activities they can enjoy for a lifetime. That means between seasons, during breaks, or even while on vacation, set expectations that your child will *move*. That might mean running, dancing, hiking, riding a bike, swimming, jumping rope, shooting hoops, or playing tennis.

8.6 CARRYOVER SPORTS

I'm a strong proponent of kids learning to enjoy physical activities they can carry over and relish for a lifetime. And I'm especially fond of those activities you can enjoy together as a family.

I remember one Halloween when Hunter was about six. We were up against the time limit allotted for our neighborhood's trick-or-treat festivities. It was 8:25, but we were compelled to visit just one more house. As we scuttled our way up the O'Learys' long, wooded driveway, we stopped short. Their lit-up family room came into view.

It appeared they were having a full-on family dance party. All five of them—mom, dad, and three kiddos (ranging from four to thirteen)—were literally rockin' out to their favorite dance music. We just stood in the dark for a few minutes, in awe, before hightailing it back down the driveway toward home. While you can bet the other neighborhood kids were sorting out their sack of sugared-up treasures, the O'Learys were in full-face-grin mode, just enjoying their family's exercise ritual. Turns out, they rocked it out like that several times a week. Is *that* cool, or what?

Our family's favorite activities were downhill skiing, backcountry camping (hiking with packs on our backs), running, and cycling. I'm celebrating that right now as I prepare to join Hunter (now twenty-seven) and his girlfriend who will guide my raft through a week of whitewater (and camping) along the middle fork of Idaho's Salmon River next week. #FeelingBlessed that, beyond his success in competitive sports, I continue to enjoy recreational skiing, hiking, and camping with him.

Think about choosing a new family activity and learning it *together*. Here are some ideas to consider:

- Camping/hiking/walking
- Yoga
- Taekwondo, jujitsu, or another of the martial arts
- Running or run-walking (consider some 5k fun runs)
- Bicycling, road touring, or mountain biking
- Tennis, pickleball, racquetball, or squash
- Swimming (pool or lake)
- Triathlons of various types and distances
- Canoeing, kayaking, or stand-up boarding
- Snow riding (cross-country skiing, downhill skiing, or snowboarding)
- Snowshoeing or skating
- Snorkeling or scuba diving
- Golf
- Volleyball or badminton in your own backyard

If you just built a mental wish list that was rudely interrupted by menacing money signs, I totally get it. Activities like golf, kayaking, or skiing might not be in your family budget right now. But when it makes good sense, consider your wish as an all-in family endeavor. You might consider replacing your family's array of holiday gifts with an investment in a new family activity. You will not regret that.

Reflecting back on my years with Hunter at home, I can remember *no* material gift or inanimate object that comes close to the specialness of our outdoor family experiences!

8.7 SPIRITUALITY THROUGH PHYSICAL ACTIVITY

Helping children find their passion and develop a sense of purpose can sometimes come from exercise, especially if they can connect to nature at the same time.

In a recent conversation with Hunter, he told me about an indelible message he received from a fellow wilderness guide, a spirit guide, he has come to call his friend: "We're continually searching for the place where our hearts first opened."

In response, I asked Hunter if he knew where *his* heart first opened, and he said, "On my first bicycle. I suddenly had such a sense of independence, like I could go *anywhere* and explore *everything*." He still LOVES cycling, especially mountain biking, with a passion.

For me, my heart first opened when I experienced snow gliding underneath my skis for the first time. I was in fifth grade and a guest of my elementary school ski club, organized by my girlfriend's mom. I was inspired by that same unbelievably free feeling, as well as the beauty around me. After that, I never stopped striving (and saving my money) for the very next time I could ski. In the eighth grade, I started spending a lot of my free time on my own skis that I bought inexpensively at a local ski swap.

My nephew Michael described that same heart-soaring feeling from running cross-country for the first time. He said, "I still love the freedom and sense of exploration I get from running, and even more now because I live in the mountains. If I'm curious about what's behind that brush, I can just run right over there and check it out."

Next is the emotional impact of movement. To me, exercise seems like a great elixir for *whatever* your body needs: If you're anxious, it calms you down; if you're sluggish, it perks you up; if you're hungry, it curbs your appetite; and if you're full, it lightens you.

As important as building physical strength for your kiddos, exercise is proven to reduce depression and anxiety while it elevates mood, cognitive function, and overall self-esteem. That's true not just for our kids, but for *all* of us.

Hunter called me recently, just to say hello. He commented that I didn't sound like myself, and I confided in him that I was feeling a little blue. Instead of asking *why*, he asked, "What are you doing right now, Mom?"

I told him I was just sitting in front of the fire, trying hard to get some work done. Then he suggested, "How about going outside for a walk, *right now*—and take me with you. I'll hang on, while you get ready." He was absolutely right. A few minutes of physical movement along with connection to the great outdoors was a powerful mood elevator.

8.8 OVERCOMING OBSTACLES

Many children will not excel in the traditional sports arena. By definition, *half* will have below-average ability—that's just life. But what if your child has physical, cognitive, or emotional challenges? Their obstacle(s) might range from simple shyness with a lack of competitive spirit to major physical disability. And the dilemma is, will this early exposure to an atmosphere of natural comparison strengthen their character? Or will it prove to be harmful to their confidence?

If you choose to enroll them, stand back and watch. As other kids notice their differences, they tend to speak up. That doesn't make them mean, just socially immature. Keep in mind your child doesn't always need rescuing because, let's face it, we're all wired for some struggle. But stay curious, especially if he or she becomes resistant or defiant about going to practice.

> Next is the **emotional impact** of
>
> *movement.*
>
> To me, exercise seems like a **great elixir** for whatever your body needs:
>
> If you're **anxious**, it **calms** you down; if you're **sluggish**, it **perks** you up; if you're **hungry**, it **curbs your appetite**; and if you're full, **it lightens you.**

Just as organized sports can boost self-esteem for some kids, it can destroy it for others. Don't let your child become the subject of continual teasing for developmental challenges that are clearly not in their control. My concern right now is not just the emotional scars it can leave. It's also that those early negative experiences might thwart their desire to explore the myriad of other physical activities that would otherwise keep them healthy throughout life.

Here's an example from my family. My brother Jim had an eyesight incapacity that robbed his depth perception. That made all traditional ball sports difficult, even somewhat dangerous. (I remember him catching a baseball with his face a couple times. It wasn't pretty!) On top of that, his physical coordination came later in life, so running and jumping sports were not his gig either. Lucky for Jim, my dad exposed us to a bunch of nontraditional sports like lake swimming, sailing, iceboating, and waterskiing. He excelled at all of them.

At the age of eight, Jim's heart came alive with waterskiing. We first learned to ski behind a little fishing boat (with a fifty-horse-power outboard motor) that my dad kept at his friend's dock. Mark, Jim, and I all enjoyed waterskiing ... but Jim LOVED it. It's a strenuous sport, for both cardio and strength, and it was perfect for him because it didn't require any physical compensations. At sixty-two, Jim is still an expert slalom skier. It's a joy to watch him! By the way, he's also a daily runner, swimmer, cyclist, and strength trainer, depending on the morning.

When I asked him *why* he became an everyday-exerciser—because remember, our parents weren't—he said this: "For me it happened as an adult, and it was all about waterskiing. In the beginning of the season, I was always so darned sore and out of shape, it was grueling. So, I started working at it year-round. Then it just became a habit."

Jim's physical limitations paled in comparison to the challenges many children face. But I truly believe our gravest disabilities can become our most treasured gifts. Part of our job as Brave Parents is to get creative in helping kids find their work-around, discover their passion, and ultimately develop their craving for daily physical activity.

8.9 SOME PRACTICAL TIPS

If you have babies or toddlers at home, you might not know how to carve out time for your own exercise. My advice ... buy a baby jogger. And if you cycle, buy a bike trailer. That way you can take your kiddos with you on your daily walk, run, or ride. Incidentally, a jogger is SO much different from a stroller. Hunter enjoyed keeping me company in the jogger until he was almost five, and I think I wore out three sets of tires. I have such great memories from our time together too.

He was more competitive than me, even as a toddler, and having him with me was sometimes like having a personal coach. He would cheer me on during 5k races, shouting with gusto, "C'mon Mom, you can take this guy." Usually the runner would laugh, while I blushed uncomfortably.

My book coach, Lauren, has an exercise area in her home. Her five-year old son liked to follow her there and imitate her movements, so she invited him to be *her coach*. He makes up his own exercises for her. To his delight, she follows his demonstration. She said, "It's never the workout I intend to do. It's even better because it spurs his interest as well." I suggested they start to take turns coaching each other.

8.10 ACCOUNTABILITY PARTNERS

Sometimes we all face this nagging dilemma: You *know* it would be good for you, but you just don't *feel* like exercising today. Not because you're sick or injured, but just because you're feeling a little lazy. With the angel on one shoulder and the devil on the other, who usually wins the final vote for you?

> 66 I truly believe our gravest **disabilities** can become our most treasured gifts.
> Part of our job as *Brave Parents* is to **get creative** in helping kids find their work-around, **discover their passion**, and ultimately develop their craving for **daily physical activity**. 99

Having an *accountability partner* eliminates that entire quandary. Your mindset becomes all about showing up. For you, that might be a coach, a personal trainer, a group fitness class, or your next-door neighbor. It's someone who is counting on you to show up.

For me, it's my BFF, Vicki. She's been my constant exercise companion for thirty-six years and counting. Most of our time together has been clocked before the crack of dawn. After we had children, that became the only time that no one else could ever steal. When we first met in 1985 BC (Before Children), we had an instant connection around humor and positivity. But the depth of our friendship has grown immeasurably over the years *because* of our time together ... on the road (running), on the court (racquetball and now pickleball), or in class (high-intensity interval training (HIIT) bootcamp).

For me personally, I can't say enough about accountability partnership. (Thank you, Vicki.) I have someone who expects me to show up every day—and it makes a difference. If you want that, try looking in your own home first. Perhaps it's your partner or even your kiddo. You can be theirs, and they can be yours.

CONCLUSION

Both daily exercise and a spirit of adventure will help keep your kiddos healthy. And it's your job to help cultivate these.

From the time I was twelve, I've been a daily exerciser. I'm not saying that to boast, but to say thanks to Dr. Zapp who gave me the gift of responsibility. I learned through her that daily exercise would keep me vital, energized, happy, and away from the doctor's office and hospital.

Someday, if you've been successful as Brave Parents of your adult children, you will have given your kids *roots* and *wings*. Roots, a sense of belonging, and wings, the autonomy to chart their own course. Instilling a joyful appetite for physical activity is a necessary part of this prescription.

There is no time like today to begin your Brave Parent commitment to daily exercise.

> **"**
>
> Someday, if you've been **successful** as **Brave Parents** of your adult children, you will have given your kids *roots and wings.*
>
> **Roots**, a sense of **belonging**, and **wings**, the **autonomy** to chart their own course.
>
> Instilling a **joyful appetite** for **physical activity** is a necessary part of this *prescription.*
>
> **"**

CHAPTER 8 REFERENCES

Banfield Pet Hospital. (2016). *Banfield Pet Hospital® releases 2016 STATE OF PET health® report.* Banfield Pet Hospital. Retrieved October 11, 2021, from https://www.banfield.com/en/about-banfield/newsroom/press-releases/2016/banfield-releases-state-of-pet-health-2016-report.

Barbieri, D., & Zaccagni, L. (2013). *Strength training for children and adolescents: Benefits and risks.* Collegium antropologicum. Retrieved October 14, 2021, from https://pubmed.ncbi.nlm.nih.gov/23914510/.

CDC. (2019, May 29). *Youth physical activity guidelines.* Centers for Disease Control and Prevention. Retrieved October 11, 2021, from https://www.cdc.gov/healthyschools/physicalactivity/guidelines.htm.

Hutchinson, A. (2011). *Which comes First, cardio or weights?: Fitness myths, training truths, and other surprising discoveries from the science of Exercise.* HarperCollins.

Koch, P. (2018, September 15). *How many calories does 1lb of Muscle Burn?* BuiltLean. Retrieved October 17, 2021, from https://www.builtlean.com/muscle-burn-calories/.

Landry, B. W., & Driscoll, S. W. (2012). Physical activity in children and adolescents. *PM&R, 4*(11), 826–832. https://doi.org/10.1016/j.pmrj.2012.09.585.

NCAA. (2020, April 8). *Estimated probability of competing in college athletics.* NCAA.org - the official site of the NCAA. Retrieved October 29, 2021, from https://www.ncaa.org/about/resources/research/estimated-probability-competing-college-athletics.

Nettle, H., & Sprogis, E. (2011). Pediatric exercise. *Sports Medicine and Arthroscopy Review, 19*(1), 75–80. https://doi.org/10.1097/jsa.0b013e318209cf2b

Norris, J. (2021, June 14). *'Metabolically healthy obesity' still raises risk of disease.* Medical News Today. Retrieved October 15, 2021, from https://www.medicalnewstoday.com/articles/metabolically-healthy-obesity-still-raises-risk-of-disease.

Sato S, Basse AL, Schönke M, Chen S, Samad M, Altıntaş A, Laker RC, Dalbram E, Barrès R, Baldi P, Treebak JT, Zierath JR, Sassone-Corsi P. Time of Exercise Specifies the Impact on Muscle Metabolic Pathways and Systemic Energy Homeostasis. Cell Metab. 2019 Jul 2;30(1):92-110.e4. doi: 10.1016/j.cmet.2019.03.013. Epub 2019 Apr 18. PMID: 31006592.

Schap, T. R. E., Klukan, S. G., & Jenko, S. (2017, February 21). *The healthy eating index: How is America doing?* USDA. Retrieved October 29, 2021, from https://www.usda.gov/media/blog/2016/03/16/healthy-eating-index-how-america-doing.

WHO. (2021, June 9). *Obesity and overweight.* World Health Organization. Retrieved October 15, 2021, from https://www.who.int/news-room/fact-sheets/detail/obesity-and-overweight.

CHAPTER NINE

in closing

GIDDYUP, YOU!

Y ou've heard it said, "Life is a marathon, not a sprint." And it's true in so many regards. Unfortunately, your time of child raising will seem like a sprint when you look back at it. Especially when you consider how little of that time YOU, as your child's Brave Parent, will get to serve as their primary influencer—before they allow their peers to seize that role. Believe me, it all happens in a flash.

So, as you might have expected, I will close with an urgent call to action. In a word, it's time to *giddyup*!

You have to brave it out! That just might mean pursuing a tongue release, scrapping a pacifier, videoing a snoring problem, pitching processed foods, banning all boxed cereals, eliminating juice and sports drinks, letting your little one play in dirt, *not* begging your doc for an antibiotic, changing health care professionals when needed, enforcing the polite bite, prohibiting screens in your kiddo's bedroom, helping develop coping skills for stress, encouraging mistakes in the learning process, talking about sex, vaccinating against cancer, and expecting *daily* exercise.

None of this is easy. If it were, everyone would be doing it, and our pediatric population would be a good measure healthier. But just because it's hard doesn't mean your child doesn't deserve it. The onus is on YOU to be tough in your resolve.

I realize there's a lot to this, and you obviously can't get there overnight. Prioritize your goals based on *your* child's truths. But *don't* take your time getting started!

Remember the proven learning concepts we discussed in chapter 6 Feel and Think: your child will learn more profoundly with spaced, interleaved practice. That means you're better off making small strides toward several concepts each day rather than mastering a single concept before moving on to another.

Build a multifaceted Brave Parent Plan and share it with any other primary caregivers including other parent(s), grandparents, daycare providers, etcetera. And then ... declare! Let your kids know you mean business and that this is all, 100%, completely out of LOVE, with a sincere desire for their health and happiness.

One of my Brave Parent team members, Jean, routinely tells her kids, "I'm the meanest mom you'll ever know, so just get used to it! I'm going to say 'No' a lot."

For her children, a trip to the grocery store is a prime example. The question "Can I get this?" frequently gets a "No," but only after she reads the ingredients list and tells them why.

When I heard this, I challenged her to rephrase her repetitive meanest-mom narrative. Instead, declare: "I'm the *Bravest* Parent you'll ever know, so just get used to it!"

And now I challenge you to adopt the same motto.

Over the past thirty-six years of caring for my patients, I've been a voracious student of some extraordinarily Brave Parents. I've watched them raise their babies into remarkably wonderful and healthy adults. And as I wrote this book, I tapped into their collective wisdom. Some of the best advice I got came, indirectly, from my eighty-four-year-old patient, Neil.

" CHALLENGE

One of my *Brave Parent* team members, Jean, routinely tells her kids, "I'm the **meanest mom** you'll ever know, so just get used to it! I'm going to say **'No'** a lot."

"When I heard this, I **challenged** her to **rephrase** her repetitive meanest-mom narrative. Instead, **declare**:

"I'M THE BRAVEST PARENT YOU'LL EVER KNOW, SO JUST GET USED TO IT!"

"

I asked, "So Neil, what's your secret? What did you and Judy do, uniquely, to raise such an awesome woman as Sarah? And what would you do differently if you were starting again?"

Right off the bat, he gave the credit to his child, saying, "Sarah was incredibly patient with me. You see, I was a very *prescriptive* parent, meaning Judy and I set forth our clear expectations based on how we saw the world around us, and we expected our children to abide. But I continually reminded our kids that we'd never done this parenting thing before. We are learning as we go, and we're doing the very best we can based on what we think right now ... but believe me, we won't always get it right.

"There were times when Judy and I were too constricting and other times when we were too lenient. As we figured that out, we had opportunities to sincerely apologize and revise our expectations. And Sarah? She just gave us a lot of grace."

Neil's message is profound. There is no dress rehearsal for parenting a child ... even if you have six kids. You have to keep figuring it out along the way. He also reminded us to ...

Be bravely prescriptive. (That means STAY STONG in your resolve.) Assert your expectations and explain why. Don't be afraid to apologize. And by all means, be patient with yourself as you figure it out.

Letting our children in on the secret (that we don't have it all figured out) is letting them see us as *real* and thoughtful people. Just like seeing us apologize to others, by admitting to our kids that, while we're trying our best, we really *don't* have all the answers, we serve as wonderful role models.

When we let our children "in," so to speak, they learn the invaluable lessons of *adaptability* and *humility* by heart.

"

Be **bravely** prescriptive.
(That means **STAY STRONG**
in your resolve.)
Assert your
expectations and
explain **why**.
Don't be afraid to
apologize.
And by all means,
**be patient with
yourself**
as you figure it out.

"

Now Back to You, My Dear Brave Parent,

I see you.

By virtue of the fact that you've read this book, cover to cover, you are a *very* dedicated parent. You are carrying a HUGE responsibility, and I admire you for it.

Now I want to embolden you as an individual. While you're Brave Parenting, it's critically important that you not forsake your *own self* for your child. Take care not to stifle your own distinctive awesomeness in this journey.

Remember that *before* having a baby, there was ... YOU. And *after* raising your babies, there will be ... YOU. Don't give up your health, your playfulness, or your personal growth during your brief-ish parenting stint.

Trust me, as your kids begin to make autonomous decisions, they don't need your 100% attention. Without oversteering, you'll get *more* opportunities to commend their successes and help navigate some of their pitfalls.

Meanwhile, your kids really *do* need you to model *self-care* and *self-love*. That means continually growing your self-awareness, self-forgiveness, and self-acceptance. Why? Because you're worth it. And ... because you cannot pour from an empty vessel.

Think about this mantra: I give "my all" to my kids. When you say that (or even think it), you subtly tell your children that it's okay for parents to forsake their OWN health for that of their children.

Part of being a Brave Parent is—get this—to parent *yourself* along the way. Commit to better health habits right along with your kids. Keep learning together. Celebrate the triumphs and grapple with challenges ... out loud and *together*.

Cultivate your support system among the other adults who love your children. And, by all means, stay connected to other Brave Parents. Together we're stronger.

"Meanwhile, your kids really do
need you to model
self-care and **self-love**.
That means continually growing
your self-**awareness**, self-
forgiveness, and self-
acceptance.
Why? Because

you're worth it.

And... because you cannot pour
from an empty vessel. "

We need to bolster each other when the going gets tough—when we're seeking some fresh, like-valued perspectives. We also need to share our success stories and get some praise from Brave Parents who "get it."

Finally, it's *up to us* to spread the word. I truly believe it's the only way we can turn our country's heartbreaking health crisis upside down. Here's an idea: if you loved this book, give copies to the parents of your kiddo's best friends. Wouldn't it be nice if these concepts became *the norm* in your child's social circle?

And with dedication, I invite you to join the Brave Parent movement. Accept my invitation on BeABraveParent.com.

I'm here to support you, with all that I am.

With love,
Dr. Susan

PS For every one of your Brave Parent efforts, your kids will thank you later. I absolutely promise that.

PPS If thanks aren't enough, your children will also grow up to live out your legacy, perhaps becoming Brave Parents themselves someday. That's when you get to be a Brave Grandparent! Life is a wondrous expedition ... enjoy the ride.

acknowledgments

I have a heart full of gratitude for so many who contributed to my life, my understanding, and my contributions.

I want to first thank my most significant teachers along my journey, my thousands of young patients and their parents. I also appreciate their allowing me to tell their personal stories.

I'm equally grateful to my team members (over thirty-six years) who have treated "our" kids like their own. They have trusted my leadership in learning to foster HEALTH in unconventional practices, like providing health-related, hands-on science experiences, for *each and every* child, at *each and every* visit. They have also imparted their wisdom on to *me*, their hungriest student.

It is a significant challenge to fulfill our mission: To take *each* little person closer to optimal health, *each and every* visit. But these women, especially, have done it with passion, love, and grace: Georgette Taylor, Jean Kolar Voss, Nikki Schram, Sara Wilson, Meghan McCormick, Amy Bruntjens, Sally Johnson, Sherry Henderson, Casey Markle, Sue Merriam, Kelly Mitchell, Tori Alicea-Price, Katie Eyde, Becky MacQueen, Brenda Burtovoy, Anna Woodard, Melissa Svarc, Emily Kramer, Diane Ballard, Corri Uschuk, and Lori Crooks. And a special thanks to two people who have always (and all-ways) believed in this big mission...my personal assistant Molly Day and my dental practice partner, Dr. Tracey Epley.

Professionally, I want to recognize my mentors, who have created deficits in my learning and spurred me on to more and more!

Especially, Dr. Bob Frazer, Dr. Mark Kogut, Dr. Doug Thompson, Joan Forest, Mary Osborn, Dr. Robert Lustig, Dr. Kevin Boyd, Dr. Steve Carstensen, Dr. Peter Dawson, Dr. DeWitt Wilkerson, Dr. Michael Gelb, Dr. Howie Hindin, Dr. Soroush Zaghi, and Sharon Moore.

And if it weren't for my two twenty-five-year practice consultants, our team would never have been able to save lives at the rate we do! A huge heartfelt thanks to Terry Goss and Janis DuPratte for your love and support, always. I continually hear your voices to our team saying, "We're running out of time in this health crisis. Your work really matters!"

A newcomer in my life, Lauren Eckhardt, my book publisher (and CEO of Burning Soul Press), fed me unfettered enthusiasm and encouragement throughout the entire process of this book. While raising children of her own, she convinced me that my words needed to be engraved in every Brave Parent's thought process, not just hers. (Thank you, Lauren!)

Special thanks to my friend Rick Exline, a man with five boys who are now grown men, having children of their own. He encouragingly reminded me that I was writing this for his sons, the Brave Fathers of the world, not just the moms.

I have a heart full of gratitude to my best friends who have consistently supported my every crazy notion to save the world: my brother Jim Smallegan and my BFFs, Vicki Schiro, Jim LeTerneau, and Dr. Denise Acierno.

Also, to my awesome (and divorced) parents, Jim Smallegan and Marilyn Sylvan Thompson, both deceased, sadly. They worked *together* and, despite my health limitations, convinced me from a young age that I could do *anything* I set out to do in life, if only I wanted it badly enough. Not so coincidentally, they were both writers when they met in the newsroom of the Detroit Free Press. They each inspired me to use my written words to awaken others.

And last, but certainly not least, I thank my personal miracle worker, Dr. Roberta Zapp. You read about her in the book's introduction. In my heart of hearts, I know I would not be here to deliver this message if it weren't for her showing up in my life as my doctor (and *surrogate* Brave Parent) as an adolescent.

With a heart full of love and humility, I feel entirely blessed, and humbled by all of YOU!

brave parent glossary of abbreviations

AAAAI: American Academy of Asthma, Allergy & Immunology

AAP: American Academy of Pediatrics

AAPD: American Academy of Pediatric Dentistry

ADA: American Dental Association

AHA: American Heart Association

AHI: apnea-hypopnea index

APA: American Psychological Association

ASD: autism spectrum disorder

BLW: baby-led weaning

BPA: bisphenol A, an endocrine disruptor

C-GASP: Children's General Airway Screening Protocol by the American Dental Association

CBT: cognitive behavioral therapy

CDC: Centers for Disease Control and Prevention

CFRC: craniofacial-respiratory complex

COPD: chronic obstructive pulmonary disease

CPAP: continuous positive airway pressure

CPS: Canadian Paediatric Society

CSACI: Canadian Society of Allergy and Clinical Immunology

CSI: chronic systemic inflammation

CVD: cardiovascular disease

DII: Dietary Inflammatory Index

ECC: Early (under seventy-one months) Childhood Caries (tooth decay) Disease

ECM: early childhood malocclusion

ENT: Ear Nose and Throat physician, also known as otolaryngologist

EPA: Environmental Protection Agency

FDA: Food and Drug Administration

GI: gastrointestinal

GRAS list: foods that the US government deems "Generally Recognized as Safe"

HDLs: high-density lipoproteins, also referred to as "good cholesterol"

HFCS: high-fructose corn syrup

HPV: human papillomavirus; our most common sexually transmitted infection (STI)

HPV-OPC: oropharyngeal cancer, primarily caused by human papillomavirus

hs-CRP: high-sensitivity C-reactive protein

HST: home sleep test

IBCLC: board-certified lactation consultant

IL-1β: interleukin 1-beta

IL-4: interleukin-4

IL-6: interleukin-6

IL-10: interleukin-10

LDLs: low-density lipoproteins, also referred to as "bad cholesterol"

mandible: lower jaw

MBSR: mindfulness-based stress reduction

MM: micronutrient malnutrition

NAFLD: nonalcoholic fatty liver disease

NCDs: noncommunicable diseases

NIH: National Institutes of Health

NNSs: nonnutritive sweeteners

NSF: National Sleep Foundation

OECD: Organisation for Economic Co-operation and Development

OMD: oral myofunctional disorder; uncoordinated, under-functioning, or over-functioning muscles

OMT: oral myofunctional therapy

OSA: obstructive sleep apnea

OT: occupational therapy

patency: openness

pharynx: throat

PPIs: proton-pump inhibitors; popular and powerful anti-reflux medications

prebiotics: plant fiber

PSA tests: Prostate-Specific Antigen test

PSG: polysomnogram

PSQ: pediatric sleep questionnaire

PTSD: post-traumatic stress disorder

REM sleep: rapid eye movement phase of sleeping

RERA: respiratory effort-related arousal

RLS: restless legs syndrome

SDB: sleep-disordered breathing

SEL: social and emotional learning

SIDS: sudden infant death syndrome

SLP: speech-language pathology

SRBDs: sleep-related breathing disorders

SSBs: sugar-sweetened beverages

SSRIs: antidepressants

T&A: tonsillectomy and adenoidectomy

TMJ: temporal mandibular joint

TNF-α: tumor necrosis factor-alpha

UARS: upper airway resistance syndrome

WHO: World Health Organization

about the author

Dr. Susan Maples is a practicing dentist, health educator, and keynote speaker. She is the author of *BlabberMouth: 77 Secrets Only Your Mouth Can Tell You to Live a Healthier, Happier, Sexier Life* and originator of the children's Hands-On Learning Lab™, selfscreen.net, and Total Health Academy. Susan is also an avid runner, walker, strength trainer, cyclist, snow skier, snowboarder, and ... sleeper. She loves to cook healthy foods, entertain good conversationalists, see the best in others, and laugh ... a lot.

www.beabraveparent.com

Instagram: @BeaBraveParent
Facebook: @BeaBraveParent @SusanMaplesDDS

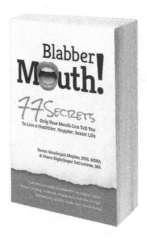

Blabber Mouth! 77 Secrets Only Your Mouth Can Tell You To Live a
Healthier, Happier, Sexier Life

CPSIA information can be obtained
at www.ICGtesting.com
Printed in the USA
LVHW081645030322
712560LV00003B/153